OUT OF THE SHADOW OF LEPROSY

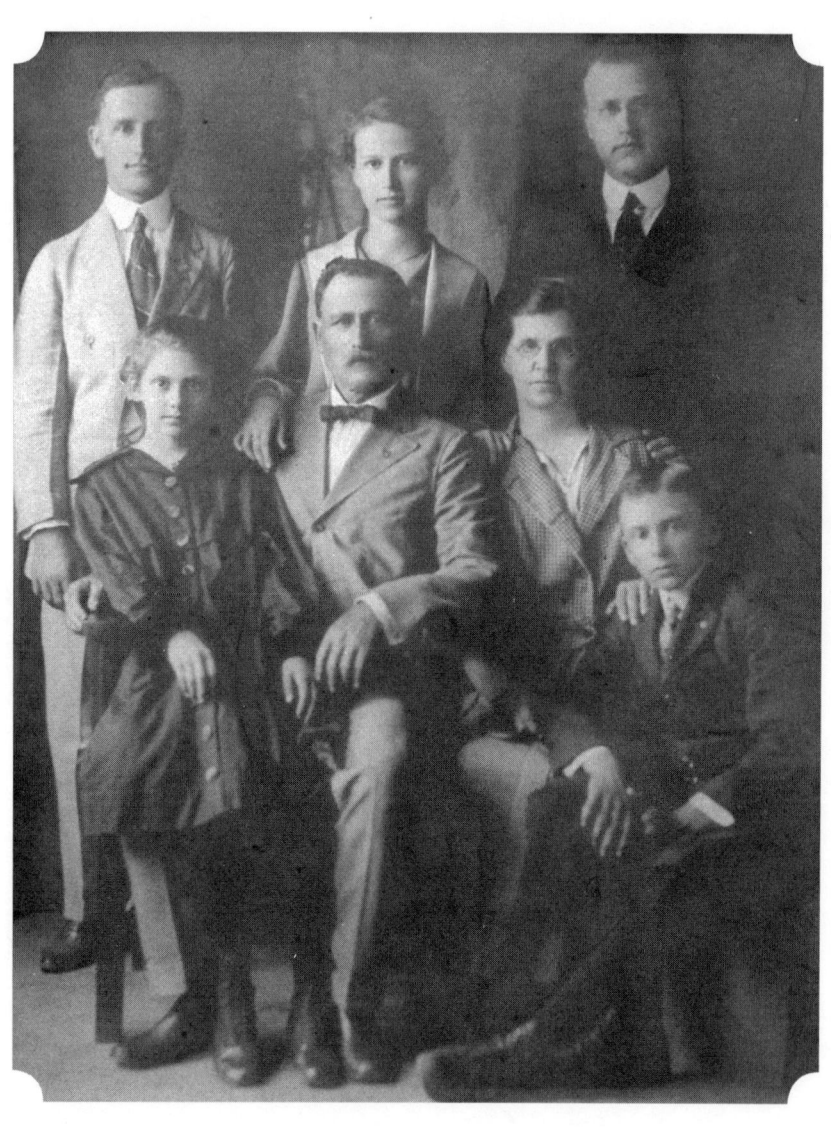

Out of the Shadow of Leprosy

The Carville Letters and Stories of the Landry Family

Claire Manes

UNIVERSITY PRESS OF MISSISSIPPI

JACKSON

www.upress.state.ms.us

The University Press of Mississippi is a member of the Association of American University Presses.

First printing 2013

∞

Library of Congress Cataloging-in-Publication Data

Manes, Claire, 1943–

  Out of the shadow of leprosy : the Carville letters and stories of the
Landry family / Claire Manes.
      pages cm
  Includes biographical information on Edmond Landry and correspon-
dence, mostly his.
  Includes bibliographical references and index.
  ISBN 978-1-61703-776-4 (cloth : alk. paper) — ISBN 978-1-61703-777-1
(ebook) 1. Landry, Edmond, 1891–1932. 2. Landry Family. 3. Leprosy—
Patients—Louisiana—Carville—Correspondence. 4. Leprosy—Hos-
pitals—Louisiana—Carville—History—Sources. 5. National Hansen's
Disease Programs (U.S.)—History. I. Landry, Edmond, 1891–1932. II.
Title.
  RC154.5.L8C387 2013
  614.5'460976344—dc23   2012036089

British Library Cataloging-in-Publication Data available

Contents

Foreword

Hansen's disease (HD) activist Stanley Stein wrote, "It is not what we have lost that matters most, but what we choose to do with what we have left." Stein entered the U.S. Public Health Service Hospital in Carville as a patient in 1931. He went on to establish Carville's international news magazine, *The Star*, and to lead the first organized patient advocate group for a disease. In his autobiography, *Alone No Longer*, Stein credits another patient, Gabe Michael, with inspiring him to become an outspoken voice for patients' rights. Gabe Michael had founded the Patients' Canteen in 1925 and the "What Cheer Club," which would eventually become the Patients' Federation. Though he died the year after Stein entered Carville, his altruism and untimely death were turning points for Stein. I knew the name Gabe Michael from Stein's book, but I did not know the personal history behind his incredible story. Nor did I know his real name (Edmond G. Landry) or his daughter's name (Leonide Landry Manes) until many years later.

My first acquaintance with the Manes family was with Chris Manes, a student worker in the English Department at the University of Louisiana at Lafayette. One day in 1998, Chris came to my office and asked if he could close the door. Then, behind the closed door, he told me that he had overheard a conversation I had had the day before. He apologized for eavesdropping, but said that he couldn't help listening. My article on the Mardi Gras at Carville had just been published in *Journal of American Folklore*, and I was talking with a colleague about my work with residents at the National Hansen's Disease Center in Carville, Louisiana. Chris then told me that his great-grandfather, Edmond Landry, had been a patient at Carville. He had died at Carville in 1932, almost fifty years before Chris was born. All four of his great-grandfather's siblings had been patients as well—members of the Landry family from New Iberia. From 1919 to 1977, one or more of the Landry siblings were patients at Carville.

Shortly thereafter, I received a phone call and visit from Claire Manes, Chris's aunt. Neither had ever spoken openly in public about their family's connection with Carville. Claire had no personal memory of her grandfather, who died thirteen years before she was born, but she had memories of his younger siblings and very loving memories of her grandmother and Edmond's widow, Claire Landry, who had lived near the Manes family until her death. She could not recall, however, her grandmother ever talking about her grandfather as a patient at Carville. She did not learn of her grandfather's illness until she was nine or ten years old, and her mother seldom talked about her father's illness.

From Claire and Chris Manes I learned that Edmond Landry's "Carville name" was Gabe Michael. They also told me about the remarkable collection of letters, written from Carville by Edmond Landry and his brother Norbert Landry, that had been rediscovered by the family. The letters are forceful testimony of the daily life, the thoughts, and the anguish of leprosy patients at Carville before the term Hansen's disease was in common usage and before there was any realistic hope for a cure. The letters are a record of their communications with family members while they were coping with an active case of a stigmatizing disease. They had none of the advantages of retrospection or the experience of improvement or cure that were typical of the narratives of former HD patients I had interviewed in the 1980s and 1990s. The letters, at times raw with emotion and at times mundane, were written at a time when there was little hope that they would ever be able to leave their virtual imprisonment at Carville. Aware of the bleak prognosis, Edmond Landry was able to chronicle his fears, his hopes, his frustrations, and at times his anger at being forced to live his life removed from his wife and young children. He was also able to maintain his compassion for others, to contribute to the welfare of fellow patients, and to find some meaningful way to live his daily life in spite of the emotional and physical pain he endured.

Other families had multiple members enter Carville as patients, but none, as far as I know, have the extensive first person accounts of their experience recorded in letters from Carville that the Landry-Manes collection gives to us. It is a remarkable collection that allows readers to witness the traumatic experience of living with an illness that led to isolation from family and total rejection by society.

In *Out of the Shadow of Leprosy: The Carville Letters and Stories of the Landry Family*, Claire Manes brings both her personal history as the granddaughter of HD patient Edmond Landry/Gabe Michael and her outstanding ability as a scholar to the fore. She gives us both the insights and the immediacy of living in the shadow of a family history of leprosy that no other scholar—unrelated and objective—could possibly give.

MARCIA GAUDET

Acknowledgments

This book, the culmination of many years of searching for my grandfather, would not have been possible without the action and support of many.

I am grateful to my cousins Paul and Martin Landry for assuring that the letters were saved and organized.

I also owe thanks to my Uncle Booz and my mother Teenie, Edmond's children, who, despite their reservations, supported my brothers, cousins, and me in saving the letters and discovering our grandfather and his brothers and sisters.

My mother, Teenie, after a lifetime of silence, finally spoke freely about her memories of her father and her life without him. She gave me a grandfather by talking about the father she missed.

My grandmother always had my love and now deserves my appreciation. While I absorbed her message that talk about my grandfather was taboo, her silence fueled my curiosity, left me with a sense that this man's life deserved study, and protected my grandfather's integrity at a time when a diagnosis of leprosy could devastate.

Marcia Gaudet's own studies of Carville gave me direction and inspiration, and her respect for Carville residents reminded me that this story was worth telling. I am grateful to her for being teacher, mentor, and friend.

David Breaux, my companion, has appreciated this story from its inception, has added insights that I have valued, and has been tireless in helping with the technical elements that elude me.

Kevin McGowan, a colleague, has been generous in his interest in my book and in his willingness to proof it and offer suggestions that have helped the clarity of my work.

Elizabeth Schexnyder, at the National Hansen's Disease Museum, was always available to answer questions and direct me to further information. Her work honors the stories of those many who could have been forgotten.

Craig Gill and Katie Keene at University Press of Mississippi have nurtured this project and helped me in untold ways; so too have Anne Stascavage, Shane Gong Stewart, and Peter Tonguette.

The interest, encouragement, and enthusiasm of my friends, colleagues, and peers have been priceless and I am grateful.

Finally, on behalf of my family, particularly my mother, I value the staff of the Carville hospital (1919–1977), especially the Daughters of Charity, whose compassion for and interest in our relatives meant so much to us for so many years.

A Chronology of Edmond Landry's Life 1891-1932

1891   Edmond is born in Segura, La., near New Iberia.

1895–1907   Births of Norbert 1895, Marie 1903, Albert 1905, Amelie 1907.

1909   Edmond attends Soulé College in New Orleans, February to August; receives his diploma in August.

1917   Edmond (26) marries Claire Elizabeth Gragnon (20).

1918   Edmond and Norbert enter the army, Edmond from June to December 1918, Norbert from June 1918 to April 1919.

1919   Edmond and Claire have first child, "Teenie"; Norbert returns from France in April, enters Leprosarium in July.

1921   Edmond and Claire have their second child, "Booz"; the La. Lepers Home becomes a federal institution.

1922   Edmond's first diagnosis of leprosy; he and Claire agree to live as brother and sister.

1923   Edmond is confined to his home with leprosy.

1924   October 10—Edmond arrives in Carville.

1925   "What Cheer Club" and canteen started by February 1925; June 25—first extant letter to family.

1926   Letters indicate difficulties between Edmond and Claire.

1927   The Great Mississippi River Flood; April 28—letter to Claire requests rescue if the levee were to break; August—Edmond acknowledges that he has not made his Easter duties.

1928   February 22—writes Veterans Bureau inquiring about coverage for family if he would leave institution or die; February 29—Edmond offers to attend a meeting in New Orleans to demonstrate the effects of leprosy; March—Veterans Bureau voices concern over Edmond's despondent letter that suggests that he might abscond or take his life; March—attends the medical meeting in New Orleans and realizes the injustice of his situation; June—Edmond writes a lengthy letter to Claire begging for conjugal visits from her; August—Edmond goes to New Iberia apparently hoping to reconcile his differences with Claire.

1929   Edmond is relieved of his duties for the Boys' House.

1930   Edmond acknowledges that he has made his Easter duties.

1931   Plans a minstrel to lift the spirits of the patient body; June—meets, along with other veterans, with Sam Jones to present the needs of the hospital; helps with the first Little Theater production in Carville; offers his cottage for several parties; enjoys visits from Claire.

1932   Is in and out of the hospital for much of the year; December 3—requests that Claire be called. The call was never completed and Claire was summoned the next day by a telegram. By the time she arrived, Edmond was unconscious.

OUT OF THE SHADOW OF LEPROSY

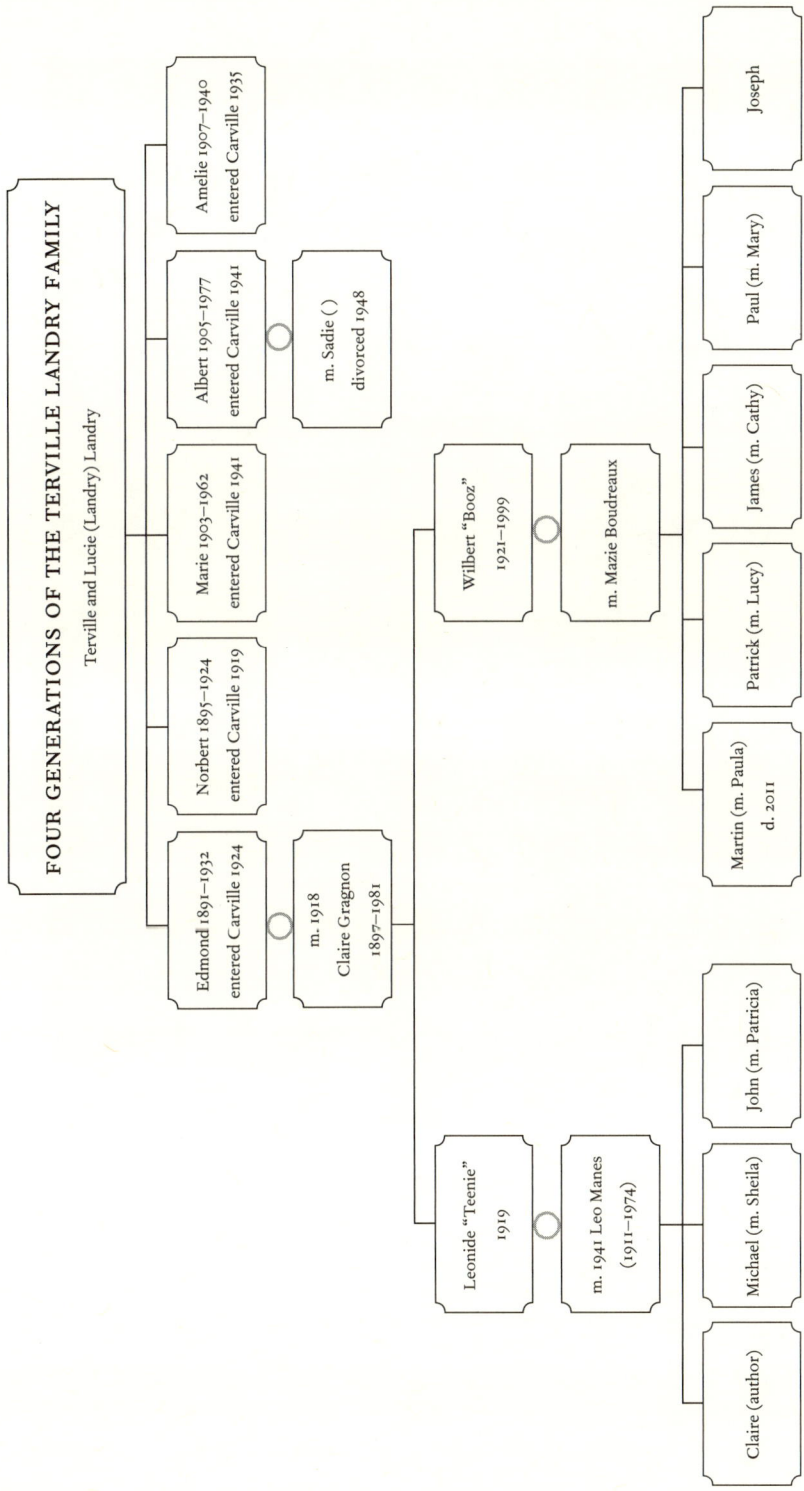

FOUR GENERATIONS OF THE TERVILLE LANDRY FAMILY

Terville and Lucie (Landry) Landry

Edmond 1891–1932
entered Carville 1924

m. 1918
Claire Gragnon
1897–1981

Norbert 1895–1924
entered Carville 1919

Marie 1903–1962
entered Carville 1941

Albert 1905–1977
entered Carville 1941

m. Sadie ( )
divorced 1948

Amelie 1907–1940
entered Carville 1935

Leonide "Teenie"
1919

m. 1941 Leo Manes
(1911–1974)

Wilbert "Booz"
1921–1999

m. Mazie Boudreaux

Claire (author)

Michael (m. Sheila)

John (m. Patricia)

Martin (m. Paula)
d. 2011

Patrick (m. Lucy)

James (m. Cathy)

Paul (m. Mary)

Joseph

Four generations of the Terville-Landry family trace Terville's children, grandchildren, and great grandchildren, the generations who lived with the sense of secrecy about their relatives.

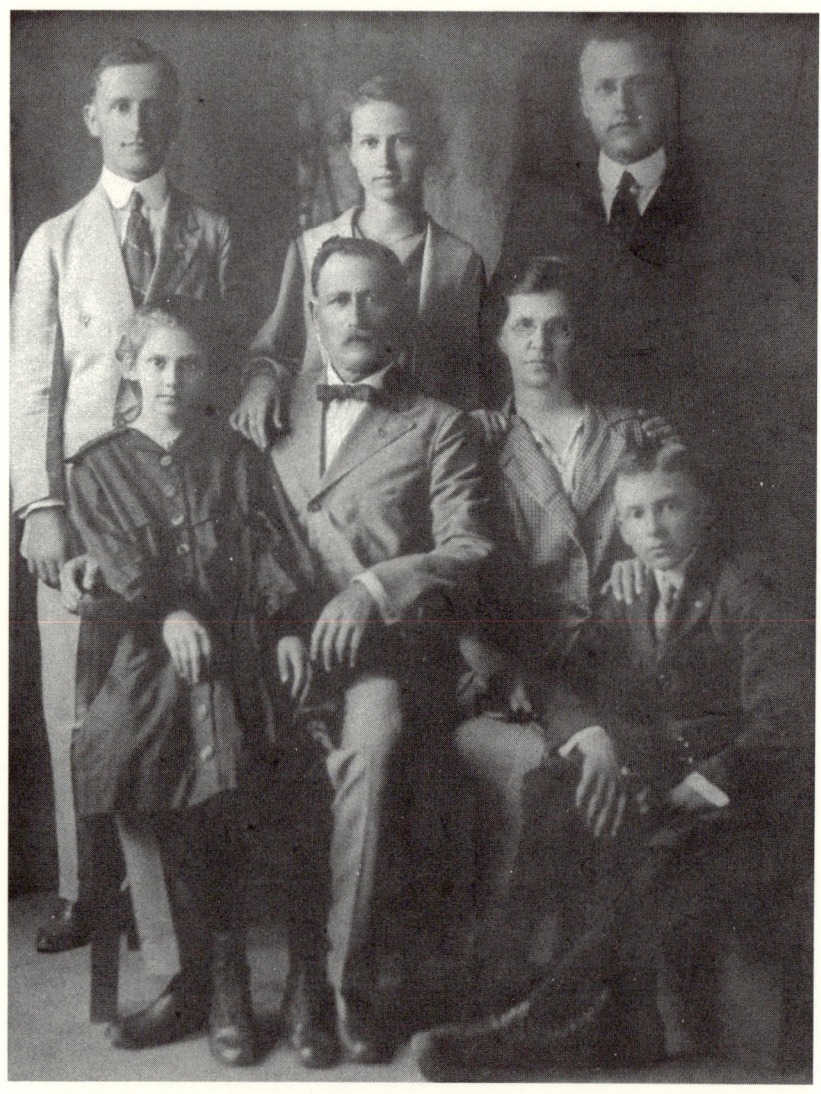

Terville and Lucie Landry (center) with their five children (clockwise from bottom right: Albert, Amelie, Norbert, Marie, and Edmond). Children are more susceptible to leprosy than adults but the disease incubates slowly. All five children may already have carried the leprosy bacillus. (ca. 1917; family collection; used with permission.)

A Family and a Disease

M y great-grandparents, Joseph Terville Landry and his wife Lucie, had five children who lived to adulthood: Edmond (my grandfather), Norbert, Marie, Albert, and Amelie. (It is believed a sixth child died in infancy.) All five of the adult children spent the last years of their lives in Carville, Louisiana, at the home/hospital for the treatment of leprosy now called Hansen's disease (HD). Norbert, the first to be diagnosed and incarcerated, was there from 1919 to 1924, followed by Edmond, 1924 to 1932; Amelie, 1934 to 1940; Marie, 1941 to 1962; and Albert, 1941 to 1977.

When Norbert was diagnosed with leprosy there was no cure for the condition, many public misconceptions about it, and little scientific understanding of its transmission. A person in Louisiana diagnosed with leprosy might hide from the public or seek treatment at the Lepers Home in Carville; there were no other viable choices at the time. The disease was mysterious, secret, incurable, and feared. Only three months after Norbert returned home from serving in the army in France in the First World War, he was diagnosed with leprosy and went voluntarily to the Louisiana Leper Home. The family was devastated that he had this disease and believed at the time he had contracted it in France. Secrecy surrounded his incarceration. By the time Edmond went to Carville in 1924, more people in New Iberia knew of his condition, but fear still surrounded him and his disease because this was now not a condition limited to Norbert but one that affected other family members. Amelie had shown symptoms as early as 1923 but remained home until 1934, perhaps depriving herself of the limited treatment available at the time. Marie and Albert managed to keep their freedom and privacy until 1941, but they had already been emotionally, if not physically, affected by the disease. Albert moved from New Iberia,

Louisiana, perhaps to avoid the disease and its stigma, and Marie never married, conceivably fearful that she could infect others.

Much has been learned about leprosy since those early days. The myth that hands or feet fall off has been dispelled. The public now knows that leprosy is a disease of the peripheral nervous system that also damages the skin; consequently, patients with untreated HD may lose the feeling in their extremities. Consequently, they often unknowingly injure their hands or feet, causing damage and deformity and possibly medically necessary amputations.

Hansen's disease is not, as long supposed, the leprosy described in the Book of Leviticus in the Bible. This biblical leprosy included multiple skin conditions that marked a person as unclean and banned from the community. This misunderstanding has led to the assumption that HD patients are somehow morally responsible for their condition and thus should remain outside the community. Even today I have heard sermons associating the leprosy in the Bible with today's HD and using the occasion to give graphic misrepresentations of leprosy, a disease like any other. Some of these sermons have been so graphic that my mother, Edmond's daughter "Teenie," has remarked that those were the only times she wanted to leave church and have a drink.

There are theories but no definitive understanding of the cause for HD. Some think that soil may hold the bacillus and there are studies linking its transmission to the armadillo. It is thought to be spread to humans by long-term association with an infected person either through skin-to-skin contact or through the respiratory system. Although we are not sure of its transmission, we do know that it is only mildly contagious. Genome research lets us know that only 5 percent of the population has a genetic predisposition to HD and even those individuals are not necessarily infected since long-term exposure to a person with untreated HD is needed to contract the condition.

It would seem that heredity would be a factor in the disease. This has not been proved, but a genetic susceptibility to it may be inherited. While all five of the Landry siblings contracted the disease, their parents showed no signs of it nor did Edmond's wife, children, or grandchildren. The same is true of other families who have had family members with the disease. One or more family members might have Hansen's disease while others are not affected.

When the Landry siblings went to Carville there was no known cure for the condition. It did not kill and it might go into remission or seem to disappear, but it was never cured. People did not die of leprosy; they lived with it in Carville. Beginning with the discovery of sulfone drugs in the 1940s and now a cocktail of three drugs, a "multi-drug therapy," people are cured of this disease in some cases in a matter of weeks. Even advanced cases that have been left untreated for a long period can become noninfectious within nine to twelve months. (For a synthesis of expert answers about leprosy, see Ramirez, *Squint* 207-214.)

In 1919, when Norbert Landry first went to Carville, none of this had been established. The family was no doubt concerned and confused by this bacillus that had entered their home. A letter from Norbert's godmother to the Daughters of Charity who were treating him perhaps says it best: "Oh please Sister, pray for us." Fortified by prayer, secrecy, and their love, the Landry family, like others with this same condition, lived for years under the stigma of leprosy. Knowledge, letters, and communication finally rescued the stories of Edmond, Norbert, Marie, Albert, and Amelie from their darkness. This book is primarily about the oldest Landry son, my grandfather, Edmond Gilbert Landry. Edmond's letters and this book are an attempt to shed light on those who have lived with HD and to bring my family out of the shadow of leprosy.

CHAPTER I

Finding Carville, Finding Family

"'At Carville' was the phrase we used to mean the disease our relatives had as well as the place they lived."
Claire Manes, author

For slightly more than one hundred years, Carville, Louisiana, a quirky village on a bend in the Mississippi River south of Baton Rouge, was an ethnic melting pot; its hospital was the home to men, women, and children from not only the United States but from locations as diverse as Japan, Puerto Rico, Mexico, and the Philippines. Those in this ethnic mix were united by the microbes that had invaded their bodies and in some cases made them outcasts from their families and themselves. From 1894–1998, Carville was home to the Louisiana Leper Home, later the United States Public Health Services Hospital #66,[1] an institution for the isolation and treatment of leprosy, now preferably called Hansen's disease.[2]

Before the home/hospital opened, patients with leprosy were pariahs, hidden away by families or consigned to pest (pestilence) houses with no hope of humane treatment much less a cure for their condition. Their disease was mistakenly linked to Biblical leprosy and thus made them vulnerable to prejudicial notions about their supposed sinfulness and lack of moral cleanliness. Because untreated leprosy could ravage the human body, deforming extremities and distorting facial features, patients could appear physically loathsome to themselves and others. Additionally, medical science knew little about the transmission and spread of the disease or its cure; consequently, the public feared, disparaged, and stigmatized leprosy patients and their families.[3]

People with leprosy were seen as exiles, the living dead. Families sometimes hid, denied, or abandoned their ill relatives. Others would drive to

8

Carville, drop off the sick, and never return to visit. Even if families did not abandon their loved ones, these patients were separated by law from spouses and children, as well as the general public. Spouses of leprosy patients could legally file for divorce. Even as late as the 1950s unwilling patients were sometimes interdicted and shackled if they refused to go willingly to the hospital. Patients from outside Louisiana were transported to New Orleans, isolated and alone in train cars, and then driven in ambulances along rough roads to Carville. In some communities, school books used by young children with leprosy were burned, and homes known to have housed leprosy patients were often abandoned, for no one cared to risk living in such environments. When the state of Louisiana first tried to institute a hospital for the care of leprosy patients, a plantation in Kenner (the planned site of the hospital) was burned because no one wanted such a place in their community. In families, stories were fabricated about missing relatives.

A friend of mine, Mary Ruth, who went to Carville in 1939, told me that she only learned that her older sister, Kitty, was in Carville when she herself was diagnosed with leprosy. Her mother had feared that the younger children knowing Kitty's whereabouts would carelessly reveal her condition to neighbors and thus bring stigma and pain upon themselves. To prevent exposure to such prejudice, Mary Ruth's mother had told her children that their older sister was at nursing school in New Orleans.

Relatives were lied about or denied, and patients were urged to change their names so as not to bring disgrace to their families. Babies born in Carville were taken at birth from their mothers and placed in foster homes or orphanages for adoption. At least one couple circumvented those rules and arranged for a nearby couple to take care of their son and daughter. Today the two children, now adults, relate stories of riding along the River Road to Carville and waiting at the "hole in the fence" for their Mamma to slip through to picnic with them on the levee.[4]

As late as the 1970s, when treatment was available, patients still experienced stigmatization. José Ramirez, a former patient and spokesperson for other Hansen's disease patients, recalls in his memoir, *Squint: My Journey with Leprosy*, that when he was diagnosed with HD and sent to Carville in 1968, Magdalena, his girlfriend and later fiancée, was discouraged, even forbidden, by her mother from continuing her relationship with him. Their love prevailed despite the fear, and they are now happily married and passionate representatives for those inflicted with the stigmatization and pain of Hansen's disease.

The pain was inordinate for those abandoned at the hospital or taken there forcibly, and even those who were visited by family felt the isolation of their condition. In the first half of the twentieth century options for release from the hospital were limited. Only a cure, rare in itself, could give a patient legitimate freedom from the hospital but not necessarily freedom from the fear of discovery.[5] The release papers indicated that the patient was a "leper" who had been a resident of the Carville hospital.[6] Patients who escaped risked a recurrence of their condition, discovery by civil or medical authorities, arrest, and a return to Carville and time in the institution's jail.

I did not know about the prejudice toward those with leprosy or the conditions of their incarceration when, as a nine-year-old child, I first repeated cruel jokes about the disease. It was at that time, however, that I learned that my grandfather had had leprosy and that his illness was a reality painful to his daughter, my mother, and a subject that was taboo to us. It was only as an adult that I became aware of the anguish, prejudice, and insufferable conditions experienced by leprosy patients and their families including my own. Even today I cannot imagine fully the pain that this stigma carried. As a child I knew I had a loving grandmother, but sensed that there was silence and an impenetrable veil of secrecy in my family about my grandfather. There were no conversations about him and no pictures of him on the wall. His life was a secret that haunted yet enticed me for much of my life.

It was at this same time that I discovered that my mother, grandmother, and great-grandmother would begin speaking French or whispering when I entered the room.[7] Context helped me to decipher some of their codes: loose smocks indicated that my mother or aunt was pregnant; glances in my direction clued me that they suspected my irritability was connected to a low-grade fever or hunger pangs. Only now in my later adulthood have I begun to surmise that some of their conversations were also about Carville, a place of mystery, the enclave of five of my relatives, and the euphemism for leprosy or Hansen's disease, which affected my grandfather and his four siblings.

Our family never spoke about my grandfather, Edmond Landry, and his siblings: Norbert, Marie, Albert, and Amelie, all of whom spent the last years of their lives in Carville at the United States Public Health Services Hospital #66.[8] We absorbed the message initiated by Edmond's wife, Claire, that questions about the family were taboo. I suspect surreptitious conversation about Carville, the place, occurred among the adults. Magazine articles and radio or television programs about leprosy may have been discussed in whispers and one time an inflamed spot on my brother's shoulder caused concern for my mother. I wonder now if Hansen's disease was feared, though my mother dismisses that assumption.

Carville, the institution,[9] was discussed, but our family in Carville was not. When my mother, in her eighties, began to talk about her memories of her father, she acknowledged, "I would probably not be talking about any of this if Mamma were still alive." Such conversation was implicitly forbidden and skillfully evaded. I remember on more than one occasion sitting in an oversized rocker in my grandmother's spacious kitchen with my mother, grandmother, and great-grandmother. I would rock and ask casually, "How did grandpa die?" For some inexplicable reason, I had an idea that if I could find a satisfactory answer to his death, I would have entrée to other questions about this man who was a mystery in my life. The mantra-like answer that I received was always the same, "He died in a hospital of a kidney disease." That answer, though true, did not satisfy me. Rather than opening conversation, the answer stifled any further questions, but it did not suppress my curiosity. Years later, when I asked my mother about those brief, rapid interchanges, she admitted, "I probably said that so you would not ask any more questions." It worked; I did not ask any more questions, but I did not stop looking for my grandfather. I scavenged in the attic, rummaged through dresser drawers, and scanned books that I imagined my grandfather had read. I hoped to find some word, mark, or memento from him. I uncovered his fiddle and mandolin, and I fantasized that glass vials, beakers, and metal frames in an armoire belonged to him, but I never found any other evidence that he had existed.

Lacking any evidence of his existence and acutely conscious of the mystery that surrounded him, I internalized the message of silence and interpreted it as secrecy. It entered the very fabric of my being and became for me a secret that was mine alone. I took some quiet pleasure in this dark, distant, unknown man. I wanted to discover him but because I feared to reveal my secret, I missed opportunities to learn about him from other relatives or his peers. I recall one occasion in particular when I was in my

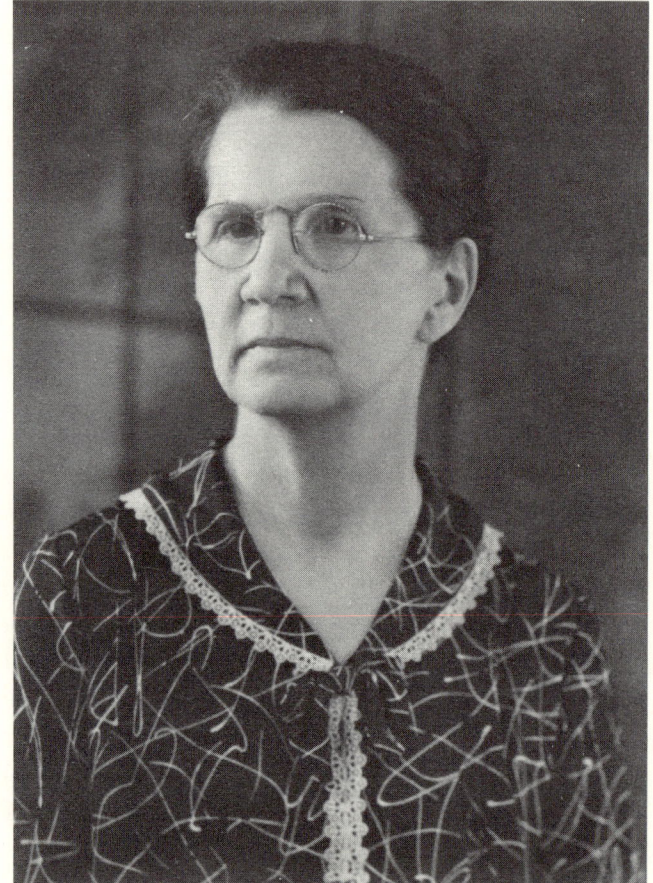

Lucie Landry kept the letters her children sent her from 1909 until she was moved to Texas in 1941. When Marie and Albert moved to Carville, they took the collection with them. (Date unknown; family collection; used with permission.)

early twenties. An older religious woman, a Sister of Mount Carmel who had been a contemporary and friend of my grandfather, began speaking about him and Val, my grandfather's good friend who was also a patient in Carville for a time. I sensed that this woman, Mother Dolores, would have told me more but coveting my secret and my sense of ownership of it, I did not pursue the conversation.

There were others who knew my grandfather, his siblings, and the family's "public secret."[10] The New Iberia postmaster, Dessard Broussard, and his wife were close personal friends of my grandmother. In his work, Mr. Dessard would have handled the family mail to and from Carville and thus would have known about my grandfather's condition even if my grandmother did not speak about it. The neighbors across the street from my grandmother knew of her husband's illness and others in the neighborhood knew he had a "bad disease." Perhaps the most touching account of public knowledge was shared with me by Peggy, my mother's lifelong friend. Peggy grew up with my mother, attended school with her, and ate many meals around the table at my grandmother's. I asked her if she had known that my grandfather had had leprosy and if that had made any difference in her friendship with my mother. Her answer was simply, "Well, there was talk, but she was my friend."

All of these incidents confirm for me that narrative evidence of my grandfather was readily available, but I identified with the family edict and held tightly to it. I indeed lived "in the shadow of what I did not know."[11] My family's secret enveloped me and I stayed trapped in its darkness, identifying with authors who held family secrets of their own. I found a certain satisfaction reading about others who searched for lost, forgotten, or denied family members. I carried traces of my grandfather's DNA and genetic makeup in my being, but I had no stories or memories of him.

Darkness would have shrouded him and his siblings permanently except for the fortuitous discovery and rescue of family letters after the death of Edmond's brother, Albert, in Carville in October 1977. When Edmond's son and daughter, "Booz" and "Teenie," and Booz's son, Paul, went to Carville to recover Albert's effects after his death, they knew about his Oldsmobile, television, clothes, and perhaps other personal items, but they were not prepared for the contents of his closet where they discovered boxes crammed with letters and mementos from the family. The collection had probably been saved by Lucie, Edmond's mother, and brought to Carville by Marie and Albert in 1941 when they, the last of the siblings to enter Carville, relocated their mother to Texas and closed the family home on Spanish Lake outside of New Iberia. My Uncle Booz and my mother, who knew their mother's fear of leprosy and were sensitive to her silence, were inclined to destroy the letters, burn them perhaps. Paul, two generations removed from the early stigma of leprosy but deeply interested in knowing his grandfather's life, prevailed upon them to save the collection. Surprisingly, Teenie and Booz agreed, despite the later protestations of their mother who said, "You're not going to keep all of that stuff are you?" The full collection, organized by Martin Landry, Edmond's second grandson, included letters from Edmond at Soulé Business College in 1909, in the army in 1918, and in Carville from 1924–1932, as well as those from

Norbert from the army, 1918–1919, and from Carville, 1919–1924. The collection had been found and organized in 1977 but read little until the 1990s, several years after the 1981 death of my grandmother, Edmond's wife. Then they were read in earnest by some of Edmond's grandchildren and great-grandchildren who irrevocably freed the correspondents from their paper prison.

Although the Landry collection[12] is incomplete, the extant letters, especially those from Edmond and Norbert, opened a window into the lives of my family. They gave me an understanding of Edmond's experiences as a student at Soulé, in the army, and in Carville. The collection also gave me insight into Norbert's time in the service, from 1918–1919, and his life as a patient at both the Louisiana Leper Home, from 1919–1921, and the United States Public Health Services Hospital, from 1921–1924. Because of the letters, I know my grandfather as a man of drive and determination, and I am introduced to my Uncle Norbert, a young man with an intense desire to reach Europe to get the Kaiser. I learned, too, of their contrasting reactions to incarceration in Carville. I can appreciate Norbert's unfailing religious faith and hope during his years in Carville, even as I suffer for my grandfather, plagued by a dark sense of injustice at his needless incarceration and his isolation from his family. The letters do not give me or any reader a limitless vista on Edmond or Norbert or on life in Carville, but they do give me insight into their lives, a touchstone for my own life, and a reprieve from the silence and heaviness that haunted me for so many years. My grandfather's letters, which are part of that collection, form the primary basis for this book: a study of my grandfather, living with integrity not the life he would have chosen but the life that was dealt him.

Because I learned about the letters at a time of transition in my own life, I did not read them immediately. In fact, I waited twenty years before I even began to study them. When I first sat with the heavy blue binders stuffed with the letters, I was anxious to read them, but I was not prepared for the power they held for me. I had looked for years for my grandfather, expecting to find some small indication of his existence, but here now was the man before me, on paper telling his story, revealing himself. I became engrossed in the letters and sought ways to further know this man. Graduate studies gave me the analytic tools and opportunity to read my grandfather's letters in depth and discover facets of his personality that would not have been evident in mementos from an attic. The more I read and reflected upon the letters, the more I realized that his story, particularly his experiences in Carville, had resonance even today, 80 years after his death. Questions from people who were mystified by Carville and leprosy and intrigued with my grandfather's life, impelled me to write about him as a man who maintained his integrity in a life that he did not choose.

His letters from Soulé College and the service helped me to see the man he aspired to be: driven, dedicated, and disciplined. I discovered a man of ambition and compassion who wanted to excel in his efforts but who could also demonstrate care for others. It is his letters from Carville, however, that show the measure of the man. Carville and leprosy forged my grandfather as the traits he had displayed earlier both sustained and tortured him in his incarceration.

New Orleans, La Feb. 2, 1909.

Mr J. T. Landry.
    Segura, La.

Dear Farther:— I entered school yesterday, I like it
very much, and I don't find it very hard I have a
very nice partner Laurent Dantervig we are in the same class
wishing to get ahead of each other.
    I am rooming with Fav; I very satisfied with this place
the lady is very nice to us all, and treats us impartially.
While at school to day I with draw a letter for
Leonce, I send it with this letter so when you see him
turn it over to him. From what I here at schools he was
not half through, but don't mention it to anybody.
Please go at Plutey and tell him to mail my
watch to 1219 Coliseum, when ready it will save
me a card and stamp.
    You can ship my typewriter C. O. D. Mr. Soule says with
typewriter you can get a much better position it would
cost me four dollars extra at school, but here it will cost
nothing.
    I am feeling well. Give best regard to all.
                    Your devoted Son,
                        E. G. Landry.
                        1219 Coliseum,
                        New Orleans, La.

(over

In his first letter to his family from college, Edmond expressed his determination to work hard to reach his goals. (Landry Letters from Carville, LLC; used with permission of the family.)

CHAPTER 2

Edmond: Anticipating a Bright Future

Soulé Business College

> *Dear Father:—'—I entered school yesterday I like it very much and I don't find*
> *it very hard, I have a very nice partner, Laurent Dauterive, we are in the same*
> *class working to get ahead of each other.*
> Edmond to his family, February 2, 1909[2]

At the end of January 1909, Edmond G. Landry left his home and family to begin his business studies in New Orleans. His trunk was packed and loaded in the buggy. He embraced his father, mother, and brother, Norbert, and kissed his younger siblings Marie, Albert, and Amelie. He left, a brash young man in a hurry. Only seventeen when he left his family for the first time, he boarded the train to New Orleans where he first resided at 1219 Coliseum Street at Mrs. Thibodaux's home and enrolled in Soulé Business College.

He began his classes on February 1, 1909, anxious to move from class to class, to complete as fast as he could the lessons that would earn him his diploma. He competed constantly, measuring himself against cousins who had not finished the program and against classmates whose penmanship was better than his but whom he could match in math. "Dauterive and I are in the same class working hard to change department this month. He is the best penman in our room, I am about medium, but am improving rapidly on penmanship practice" (February 7, 1909). Bahon,[3] a student ahead of Edmond who worked faster than he, was his particular rival. "I am working hard to make up my average and I would give anything to beat Bahon as Verret I beat twice already" (May 1, 1909). Finally, on May 23 Edmond achieved his goal: "I at last did what I had been working for, I beat Bahon on the last exam 10 points so far as Verret and Daut I got them beat on the general average, but Bahon has me beat a few points on the general average" (May 23, 1909, to Norbert).

Initially, he took little time off, as he admitted, "I have not gone out at all since I am here, the only place that I went is to school and to church, for I am studying hard to get out of that room that I am in before next month" (February 19, 1909, to Mother). He rued time missed from school for holidays because this only prolonged the time spent in school later and ultimately hampered him from his goal of completing his program as quickly as possible. "I am certainly angry of those holidays [probably Mardi Gras] for it puts us back a great deal for we have to have one thing verified before starting another" (February 19, 1909, to Mother). As he advanced in the program, however, he became more relaxed and took time off to visit New Iberia, go to the races, and spend time with friends in New Orleans, enjoying good food, music, and the company of the young women whom he met. "There is one of my old girl friends that is going to school at Soulé that I met at Aunt Lou's it is Jouliet Jolisant one of aunt Marie's old friend's daughter" (February 19, 1909, to Mother). A return to New Orleans after a weekend home in New Iberia offered further opportunity for socializing. Edmond tells his mother in a June 25 letter, "We were together as far as Franklin coming back, for Daut did not come back that night and Verret was with a girl so I thought I would stay with them, she seem to be very nice, she said that I had to come over and meet her little sister, so I thought I would, well I went but when I got there I found out that her little sister was a big sixteen year old and not at all ugly; she is the picture of Alexine Colgin. I spent a nice evening, heard some nice singing and music, and they treated me very nice and even invited me to come over any time [to] take dinner with them."

The school's demands appealed to Edmond and shaped the focus and discipline that remained with him for the rest of his life. He took courses in math, bookkeeping, and commercial law, and had tests at least two or three times a week. He had his typewriter[4] shipped from home and taught himself to type to avoid the school's $4.00 typing fee and because skills in typing could bring a better salary. He also spent time working in the school's office and commercial banking programs where he gained experience as a bookkeeper, bank manager, and bank president. He especially loved the practical experience this gave him and wished he could have spent more

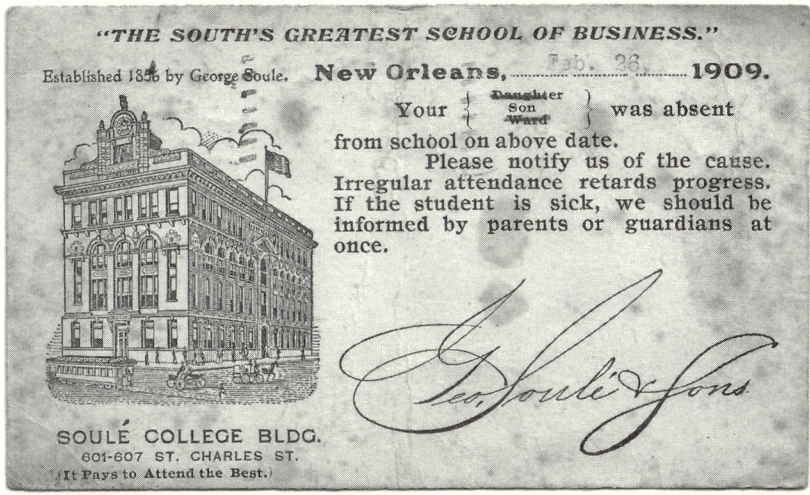

Edmond's father was sent an absentee report when his son missed school. (Family collection; used with permission.)

time in that segment of the program. "I am in the office this week representing bookkeeper for D. D. Ewing, of Memphis, Tenn., that's one week's work for day and night school, I went to school Saturday for explanation of the office work, it seems to be very nice, and is exactly as if you were keeping books in a real store. . . . I have but two more sets to work before taking up banking, that's the time, you have to handle 27 books at one time; the most I have handled at one time till now is 8, I am now keeping books for a Plantation it is very simple" (May 17, 1909, to Father). To his brother, Norbert, on May 23, he added, "I am finishing my week's office work; I wish I could stay in the office a week longer for I am crazy about the work." And in June he noted, "I am still in the bank on my last office that is president, that's once I will be able to say I was president of a bank if it is the only time" (June 25, 1909, to Mother).

The school offered a self-paced program with students moving forward as they successfully completed the required packets. They were admonished to do their best and were reminded on the school's letterhead that "what is worth doing is worth doing well." Home study tablets for the students were emblazoned with the reminder that "faithful home study is absolutely essential to student success." Parents of absent students were sent postcards recording their son or daughter's absence and cautioning

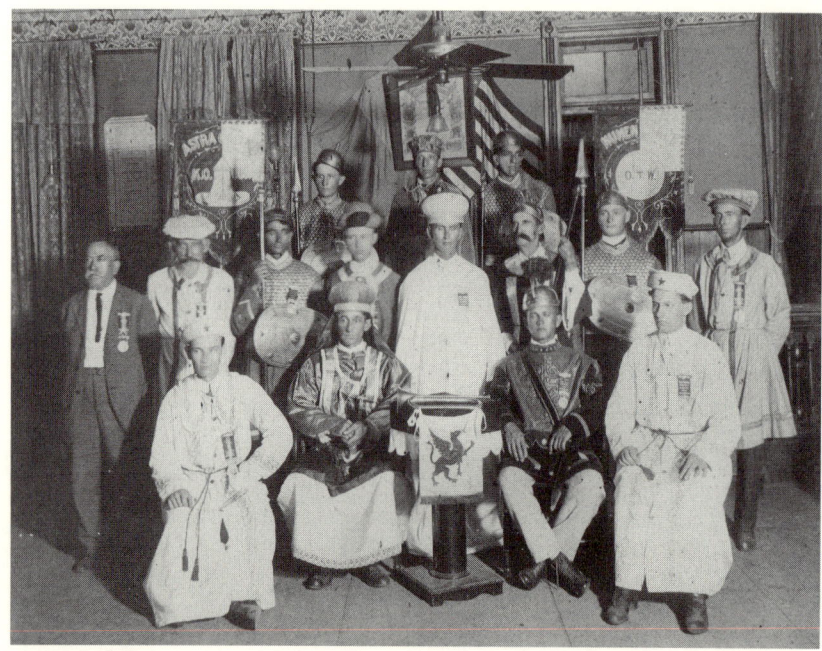

Edmond completed his program at Soulé in August 1909 and returned to New Iberia entering into the business, religious, and cultural activity of the town. At some point he joined the Knights of Pythia, a non-sectarian, fraternal order dedicated to service. (Family collection; used with permission.)

that "irregular attendance retards progress." A strict business dress code obliged male students to wear coats in the building even in the heat of summer. Partial answers in math were wrong and cheating was absolutely forbidden. Soulé's rules for arithmetic had to be followed and students had to complete complex multiplication problems instantly as they were written on the board. It was said of the students that they "majored in perfection" (Carolyn Kolb, 106).

Edmond explained the testing system to his brother Norbert in a May 23, letter. "I will have to take finals before long, but it is entirely different to yours, the average mark here is 70 but it is harder to make a 70 percent average than an 80 at public school for at the high school or elsewhere if you work a problem by the correct method and get the wrong answer you [are] getting half, but here you must work it by the right method or get zero, if the answer of a sum is 496262.04 and you get 496262.02 you get zero, if you get every problem right but you are caught talking during the examination, you will have to prove him that you were not talking about the exam, and he will give you ½ otherwise you would get zero."

Edmond's first grades for February and March were "fair," as he told his parents, but he maintained a determination to improve. He was not sick often, but when he was he usually maintained his attendance. On the other hand, on at least two occasions he missed school to study at home where he could spread out his ledgers and not be interrupted by "gumps" who distracted him with their talking or incessant questions. "I suppose you receive another postal from Col. Soulé, well I staid home to work on my book with more care and in quiet; for at school I am seating between two big 22 yr old gumps who carry on the biggest hurrah all day that it is almost impossible to do neat work, and already my work does not look so very neat on account of my writing" (May 17, 1909, to Father).

He valued education not only for himself but for others, encouraging his brothers and sisters to succeed in their pursuits. He believed that education was important for girls as well as boys and felt that his female cousin, Flavie, should be kept in school even though she had been caught writing notes to boys. "Uncle Henry caught Flavie writing to boys; he gave her a good scolding and says that he is going to take her out of school[.] I don't think he should take her out but give her a good whipping every time it happens" (March 22, 1909, to Norbert). Edmond's interest in education for his family included encouraging their efforts, even correcting letters sent to him by his sister Marie so that she could learn to improve her correspondence. While Edmond was in the army he also challenged his brother and sisters not only in schoolwork but in their music as well. "Would like for Amelie and Marie to tell me if they are studying these days. I dreamed that they were not, especially Amelie, and if they don't it is sign that they don't care to be able to play well when I get back soon.[5] Now if that is the case and they don't do better, you all better sell the piano and use the money for something else. As to Albert he had better study for when I get back I will have some work for him and [if he] does not study he won't be able to do it" (July 24, 1918, to Folks).[6]

Edmond's education was important to him, but so were good food and comfort. He missed the watermelons, strawberries, and plums from home, and he also valued the good food in New Orleans. He and his roommates moved at least twice in their six months in New Orleans, living first on Coliseum Street; then at 1016 Camp, boarding with Mrs. Barré; and finally

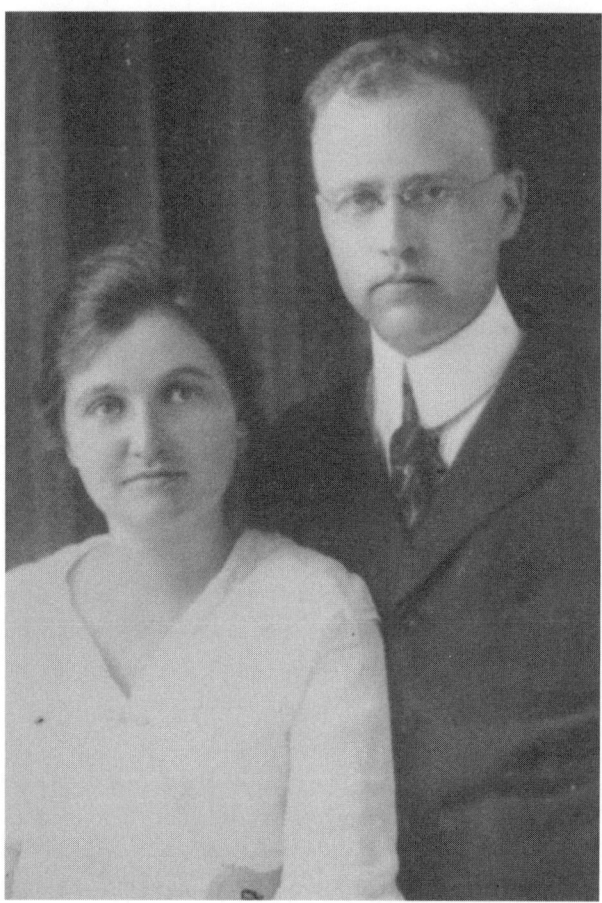

Edmond and Claire. Edmond married the only woman he ever loved in December 1917. (ca. 1917; family photo; used with permission.)

at 759 St. Charles Avenue. Each time they moved, they did so to be closer to school or for better food: "three full meals, different every day and dessert." When the young men did move, Edmond expressed concern for leaving the homeowners without boarders; however, on both occasions he was assured that they understood and complimented him on his good manners. When his friends moved to St. Charles Avenue, he waited to join them because the only room available was in the attic and too hot. "I would go too but the only vacant is one in the attic and it is hot in there as in hell for it is right next to the slate roof and the sun heat[s] those slate all day long and you know at night it must not be cool in there for they cool off only when it rains. They [presumably the meals served by the Barrés] have gotten a little better since Daut [left] for I think that they heard it was on account of the meals that Daut left and the thing that keeps me here is my room it is a big room very nice and cool and I prefer a nice and cool room to a nice dinner for any eatable will keep you up any how not fancy but I study hard and go to bed late and when I go to bed I like to sleep and you know that I can not sleep in a hot room" (May 1, 1909, to Mother).

He made the most of his schooling in New Orleans, but missed his family, cherished the letters he received from them, and chided them when the correspondence was not frequent enough. He wrote regularly except when he had major exams, and he expected that someone from home could write to him as well. He encouraged his brother Norbert and their cousins to come to New Orleans to visit. "Tell Pierre to come on the next Excursion any how alone to let me know and I will meet him at the train there is no danger of missing each other there" (May 7, 1909, to Mother). Then on July 10 he suggested to his mother, "If you think it is too hot for you to come on the next excursion try to send Norbert [who was fourteen at the time] for I know he would like to see the city, I would be able to show it all to him, if no one can come with him and if he is brave enough he can come alone as there is no danger I surely will see him try to have Simon or Pierre come with him."

He was glad that Amelie smiled when the family talked about him and he wanted to know if she was learning to walk and talk. He was concerned that Albert and Marie would remember him and he wrote encouraging letters to Norbert. He longed for his family but maintained his commitment to his schooling. He completed his program in August 1909 in the heat of the summer, six and a half months after he arrived in New Orleans. Although he finished too late to participate in the summer graduation ceremonies, he did receive his diploma. "You tell me in your last letter to buy me a frame for my diploma as I could get them cheaper down here, I could but it would not go in my trunk, but I have not gotten the diploma yet but I don't think that there is much to prevent me from getting one" (July 31, 1909, to Mother). His hope had been to finish in early August, but he was held back for a time in the last room. "Well we will all be away from here in a couple of weeks, Verret is leaving today on number 9, he got his diploma yesterday, if I would not have been held back as [I] was two weeks ago, we would all be leaving next week" (August 5, 1909, to Father). Additionally, miscalculations on his final exam made it necessary for him to repeat the test. "I suppose that you all are expecting to see me down there today or tomorrow

Camp Pike Ark
July 8, 1918.

Dear Folks:—

No doubt you all are expecting this letter as I told Claire that I would write you to-night.

I received Marie's letter to-day also one from Claire. I don't understand that you all did not get my letter that I wrote last week.

We are still in quarantine and are not doing much Yesterday was a holiday and this morning I was interpretor This afternoon was pay day for the old men so we did not drill. Getting off pretty easy so far.

While at Camp Pike in Arkansas, Edmond wrote regularly to his family and to Claire, but he also expected letters to be shared so that he could save the price of a stamp. (Landry Letters from Carville, LLC; used with permission of the family.)

but I am sorry to say that I will not be there before Tuesday, I would of gone back to morrow, if it were not for a slip I made in my calculation yesterday, in my examination which I will have to take again Monday, but you all can expect and meet me at Lafayette Tuesday. I will be down on No. 9 due at home at 4:28" (August 14, 1909, to Mother).

He left New Orleans by train for home in mid-August. His homecoming was an excuse for the entire family—parents, brothers, sisters, grandparents, aunts, and uncles—to celebrate with a family gathering and meal before Edmond officially stepped into the adult world.

The next seven years were important but unrecorded. Edmond found work in or near New Iberia, apparently as a salesman and bookkeeper for Estorge Wholesale Drug Company. In 1915 or 1916 he met Claire Elizabeth Gragnon, the woman he came to love and later marry. Claire was visiting her New Iberia relatives, the Courregés, and missed the train back to New Orleans. Edmond was one of the young people invited to visit with her while she awaited the next train. It was time well spent. Edmond and Claire were writing of their love by October 1916 and were married a year later in December of 1917, beginning a life together before Edmond departed for the service.

The Army: Camp Pike, Arkansas

Dear Mother, Father & Folks
Reached here yesterday morning as you no doubt heard from Claire.
Everything went through fine. . . . Just the shaving part that gets my goat but I guess I'll be better off when I get used to it.
Edmond's first letter to his family from the army, Saturday, June 28, 1918.

In June 1918, Edmond again left home, this time to serve in the army at Camp Pike in Arkansas. Both he and his younger brother, Norbert, served in the military, Edmond stateside and Norbert briefly in France. Their ability to speak French was an asset to them in the service. Both men could serve as translators and Edmond also wrote letters for those unable to do so themselves. "Just wrote 7 letters and they all want to give me a quarter" (Saturday, June 28, 1918, to Mother, Father, and Folks).

During his tenure in the service, Edmond chafed at the regulations, especially shaving, and he preferred giving orders rather than receiving them, which is one reason he appreciated his first promotion. "Don't know how you all found out that I was Corp[oral] but that is correct. I was appointed last Saturday. It came as a surprise for I had not put in any application for promotion. That doesn't only mean that I do the ordering instead of being ordered but it brings me $6.00 per month extra, making altogether with the Government Allotment to Claire $51.00. Could have landed a good job yesterday which would have netted me $66.00 but I was not familiar enough with the work to attempt it. They better not give me the same chance next month. So far I am tickled over my positions" (July 24, 1918, to Folks). A second promotion came in August. The August 15 letter describing his promotion also attests to his patriotism, frugality, and his demands on himself and others. "The reason that I did not write, was that I knew Claire showed you all the letter I wrote her and it was useless to waste three cents to write the same news. You no doubt realize the three cents is a large amount when you are on an army salary, drawing the pay of a private. I am glad, however, to say that I will draw the pay of Sergeant next month, which is $38.00 per. Our last pay of $36.00 for Corporal was not issued due to some errors in our transfer and it is beyond correction, so we are just out of $6.00.

"That extra $8.00 per month will come in handy, as next month will be another drive for Liberty Loan and all Soldiers, are requested to buy a Bond, if they can afford it, and of course it is hard for a man drawing more than a private's pay to get out of it, which is nothing but his duty and helping himself. If he keeps the money on himself, he will spend it for foolishness, whilst if he invests it, it will be helping in two ways, and he will not notice it." The foolishness he noted included some of the men gambling their salaries and having nothing left on payday. By contrast, he seems to have been frugal with his own funds. "I feel bad for a few uneducated Frenchmen here and there is another bunch that will feel bad before long as they shoot craps and play poker all day long and some will soon be broke. Pay day does not get here before 60 days or more. I am not worried as I have not spent but 45 cents since I left" (June 28, 1918, to Mother, Father and Folks).

He utilized the training he had received at Soulé since for much of his six months at Camp Pike he was involved in clerical service which he liked despite the fact that he had no holidays, not even Sundays. "I don't know much of what is going to be done here nor how long we will be here but I am in the office as Company Clerk for the present and hope to keep that for a while, as it is pretty easy. The only thing I don't like about it is that we have no holidays, not even Sundays" (July 20, 1918, to folks). Thus, on August 4 he wrote, "I am now at the K[nights] of C[olumbus] Club waiting for Mass to start. Had to walk fourteen blocks to get here. There is a Chapel (four blocks from our new place) but Mass there is at 9 and I was busy at that time, so had to come here or miss mass. This is where I used to attend mass."

His clerical work involved processing men arriving on the base and also made him privy to the deployment plans for soldiers in his unit. "It surely did hurt my heart to-day to have to send a few of these men across as I made up the list with the Captain. They don't know a word about it" (August 19, 1918, to Papa and Folks).

Edmond's work in the office meant that he was physically less prepared for drills. "[S]tarted drilling this week. I drill in the morning and Martin, my friend, drills in the afternoon. It is pretty hot on the drill grounds, so dam hot that this morning I had to quit. I wanted to keep on and try to hold out but one Lieutenant told me it was best for me to drop out. It is just the lack of physical exercise that caused it. You see I have been doing office work, mostly, since I am here and the other men have had three weeks exercises and drills which puts them way ahead of us and it makes it heavy work for us to hold out with them. Guess after a week's time we will be in good shape. We were at the rifle range Tuesday and my shooting is about the average" (August 15, 1918, to Papa and Folks).

Although he struggled during his first efforts on the field, he soon managed to gain the strength and discipline needed for the required physical effort and he was pleased when he passed his physical for overseas deployment. "We passed our over seas exam yesterday and I am O.K. and I am certainly glad. Not that I am glad that I will cross but glad that I am physically fit for I would hate to be turned down on account of not being all man. This over sea exam doesn't mean that we leave soon but just to classify us. . . . You know a man in the Army doesn't know where he stands, regardless of his position, from private to major, he is here today and doesn't know where he will be the next day" (August 4, 1918, to Mother and Father). By November, he had gained strength and muscle. "Am getting to be hard and a four mile hike we had yesterday just limbered me up and gave me a terrible appetite. The hike was made with a 50# pack and our rifle but I did not feel the weight at all. We also had to put up and take down tents yesterday for field inspection" (November 3, 1918, to Brother and Folks).

He took his jobs in the service seriously, but also showed concern for the Landry family's well-being. Upon entering the service, he took out a life insurance policy that listed his wife Claire and his mother as equal beneficiaries. As he explained to his mother, the arrangement was one insisted upon by Claire, who was given the power of attorney for Edmond should anything happen to him. On another occasion, he sent home a coat that could benefit his brother. "The coat I sent back was given to me and is too big for me so mamma can make a coat for Albert or save it for me when I get back" (October 27, 1918, to Marie and Folks). He expressed interest in Norbert's service experiences and also sought to assure his parents that their son was safe. "Guess you all got a letter from Norbert by now or will be getting one in the next few days. Even though you don't get any news there is no need of worrying about his not being O.K. for if he was not you would get immediate telegraphic notification. His first letter or letters may go astray and cause a very long delay. If he was on the torpedoed boat he will no doubt say so when he writes as we have received letters from a few boys saying that they were on this boat. I don't think he was he must have been a few days later" (October 6, 1918, to Folks and Claire). The success of the family farm also interested him. "I understand the cane crops are moving very rapidly. When you write next let me know the cane's average per acre, about how many tons papa expects to make and how much they are paying" (November 3, 1918, to Brother [Albert] and Folks).

His army career was short. The war ended in November 1918, and Edmond returned home in December before Christmas, ready to celebrate with his family with home cooking and cherry bounce. "It is also against the rules to have cherry bounce here. Just keep it for me when I get back and we will make up for lost time" (August 4, 1918, to Mother and Father).

Following Christmas, Edmond returned to employment with Estorge Wholesale, and he and Claire, living less than three miles from his family home, awaited the birth of their first child. Leonide Lucy, "Teenie," my mother, was born on February 19, 1919. Edmond, Claire, and Teenie had become a family.

Life for this close-knit family was not yet complete, for Norbert was not home from France. He missed the family Christmas and was not around for the birth of his niece. In particular, his mother was concerned for her second son and perhaps feared a problem with his return. Norbert did return to the United States in late April and wrote excitedly about being home in the good old U.S.A. He was briefly stationed at Camp Shelby in Mississippi before being discharged. Norbert was back in Louisiana by May, ready to see his fiancée Louise[7] and his family, and to begin work as a garage mechanic. Both brothers were working and the family was together; 1919 was now going to be a good year for the Landry family.

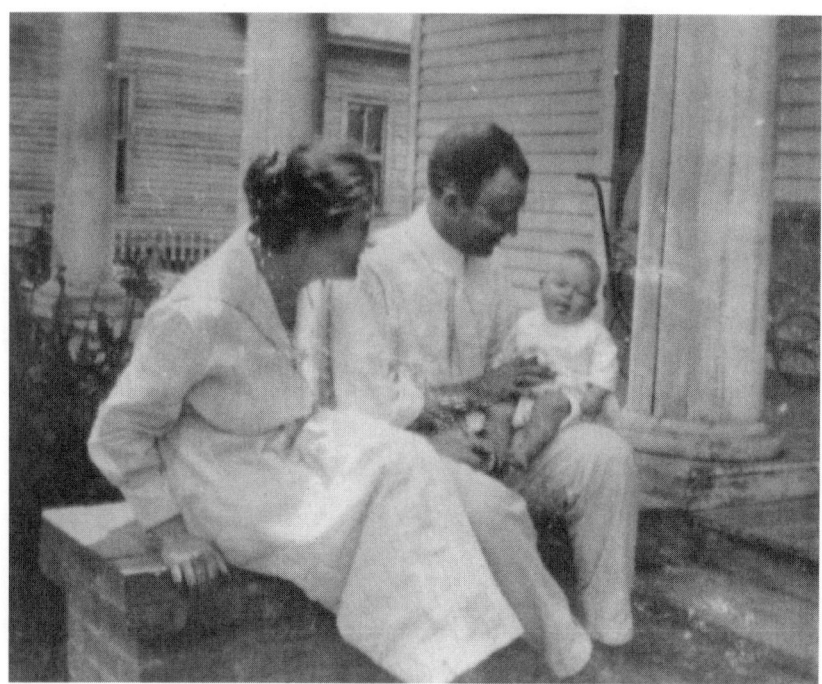

Edmond, Claire, and Teenie in the summer of 1919, a good year before leprosy invaded their life. (Family photo; used with permission.)

CHAPTER 3

Moving into the Shadow: Life at Home

"[Edmond is] a mighty-good citizen, an exemplary father and husband and valued highly by our entire community"
a letter from Dr. Carstens to Dr. Denney, October 8, 1924, hand carried by Edmond upon his entrance to Carville

My favorite picture of my grandfather is one of him, my mother, and my grandmother taken in the spring or early summer of 1919. It is my grandfather's best picture, and one that is indicative of the best years of his life. In the picture, he and his wife are sitting outside on the stoop in front of their rented home on Main Street in New Iberia. The sleeves of his white business shirt are rolled up, his tie is slightly loosened, and he is looking delightedly at his chubby young daughter, Teenie, sitting on his knee. His smile crinkles his eyes and his hands steady his daughter who, tongue out, drools contentedly. My grandmother sits by her husband; her hand brushes her daughter's leg and her attention is focused on this, her first child.

Although records now indicate that leprosy had already invaded Edmond's body, he was not hampered by that knowledge or by the disease's ravages. He was anticipating a life that balanced family, religion, and work. He was with Claire, the woman who was the answer to his prayers, and together they were raising their daughter, Teenie. The story of his life mirrored that of many other men of his generation. Family, work, and devotion to religious faith occupied his time, and his efforts at these were rewarded. Edmond and Claire were clearly content as they doted over their daughter in the spring of 1919, but even as they sat together, the specter of leprosy was upending their life.

By July 31, 1919, Norbert was at the Louisiana Leper Home in Carville, the first of his family to be confined with leprosy. He was writing letters home relating the loneliness of the place and the rituals of his religion that sustained him: Mass, rosaries, novenas, and Benediction. He told of his efforts to stay busy: hiking and hunting on the grounds, raising watermelons, watching the Home's weekly movies, painting and helping to clean around the Home. Norbert exuded a naïve optimism, believing that prayer, good hygiene, and medicine would effect a cure for him. He wrote often of the doctor's encouraging words about his condition and held out hope for a release from the hospital and a return home. He wrote home about his needs for clothing, a hat, leggings, and personal items that the Home did not always provide. In the early days of his confinement, Norbert wrote glowingly of the generosity of the Daughters of Charity, especially Sister Regina, whose solicitude eased his loneliness. Visits by the family to the Home revealed its financial difficulties, and both Edmond and his parents sent gifts to ease the strain on the Home and to add some small enjoyment to the community. They sent monetary donations as well as sheep for the sisters, a goose for the priest, small gifts of food and candy, and a little dog, "Zip," for Norbert. Norbert's letters to his family and to Edmond gave my grandfather insight into the Home and hospital. As the oldest son and the one living in town, Edmond took care of Norbert's personal and financial needs. Claire baked cakes and made candy for him, sending novenas and prayers along with the homemade treats.

Whether or not Edmond visited his brother, Norbert's letters must have caused him concern. When Norbert wrote in November 1919 that Louise had broken their engagement, Edmond may have had a pang of fear that the same fate could be his. He and Claire were married, but he knew her fear of leprosy for herself and especially for the children. Perhaps Edmond remembered the anesthetic spot on his ankle that had troubled him in 1917; surely he feared that Norbert's leprosy might be hereditary and contagious. He and Norbert had shared a room and personal effects during their childhood and adolescence. Nonetheless, he and Claire moved on with their life, buying a home on Weeks Street, raising their daughter Teenie and later their son Wilbert, "Booz," who was born in October 1921, six months before Edmond's first official diagnosis of leprosy.

My grandparents' life was tranquil between 1919 and 1922. Edmond was healthy, and he and Claire were hopeful that he would not suffer the same fate as Norbert. However, in 1922 leprosy became a personal issue for the couple when my grandfather was diagnosed with the disease. His family physician, Dr. George Sabatier, maintained progressive views on the disease and did not report Edmond to the local health authorities; to do so would have meant Edmond's incarceration in the United States Public Health Services Hospital #66, administered by the federal government since 1921.[1] Because of Dr. Sabatier's benign approach, Edmond for a time remained an active respected citizen in New Iberia, a possible mayoral candidate, and a member of the Knights of Columbus. He continued working as a bookkeeper at Estorge Drug Company. In town, he heard the speculations of others about leprosy, stories of people suspected of the condition, and curiosity about people who had mysteriously disappeared. There were idle gossip and questions about Norbert who was known to be in a Veterans' hospital but whose condition was only suspected. The effort to remain reticent about his own condition and to respect Norbert's request for secrecy strained him, but the opportunity to work and to provide for his family sustained him for another year.

However, insurmountable changes had already erupted. Claire had an inordinate fear of her husband's condition and requested that she and Edmond live as brother and sister once the diagnosis was given. She realized Norbert had been hospitalized with leprosy and now her husband was facing the same fate. Like so many others of her generation, she was ignorant of the causes of leprosy and prejudiced by false knowledge about it. She feared catching leprosy herself and feared too that their children were heirs to the disease.

The fear never left her; years later, even after treatment was discovered for the disease, she still plied her adult son and daughter with rubbing alcohol anytime they returned from visiting their Aunt Marie and Uncle Albert, who were the last of the family to reside in Carville. Her apprehension affected our generation as well, for she remained diligent of her grandchildren's actions that might in any way expose them to leprosy. My mother and her brother had by then inherited the Landry property on Spanish Lake. The family home, a wood and *bousillage* (mud and moss) structure, abandoned since 1941, still stood on the property and was a source of curiosity for us kids and of anxiety for my grandmother, who was terrified that if we explored the home we might be susceptible to the germ that had so affected the family. My grandmother's fears prevailed and the home was torn down.

Recently, medical science has noted a connection between armadillos and leprosy in humans. An April 27, 2011, article in the *Los Angeles Times* quotes Richard W. Truman, director of microbiology at the National Hansen's Disease program: "People get leprosy from these animals." My brothers and cousins spent endless hours unsuccessfully chasing the creatures in my grandmother's backyard. I am sure that had "Mamman," now deceased for 30 years, known about this theory the boys would have been banned from the chase if not the yard itself, and she would have declared war on the armadillos.

For Edmond, the 1922 diagnosis was one that he must have dreaded even as he viewed it as a trauma that seemed inevitable. There was not a definitive understanding of how leprosy was contracted, but it was at times found in families and a diagnosis, even if expected, was always "devastating" (Gaudet, 25). Despite the 1922 diagnosis, Edmond still maintained a semblance of normalcy in his life. He still lived at home; he had his children, his work, and a daily (though only companionable) relation with his wife. He and his family must have prayed for a cure, a remission, a misdiagnosis, anything that would avoid the inevitable. Rosaries and novenas were said and held at bay a final diagnosis until May 1923 when Edmond was declared totally incapacitated for work and was confined to his room at home.

No longer was he a man in charge of his life, energized by his work and loved by his family. He became, in the words of Arthur W. Frank, a member of the "remission society,"[2] one who would never again be well. More and more decisions were made not by him, but about him. He endured the terrible lethargy of a disease which could not be cured and which was considered a stigmatizing and reportable offense, subject to incarceration in the United States Public Health Services Hospital, a place that confined his brother Norbert[3] and would finally be his home as well.

Edmond was a patient/prisoner in his own room. His two children never again sat on his lap or even saw him alone but always under the nervous gaze of their mother or grandmother. His weak hands and legs crippled him, and he risked being recognized as a "leper," someone who must be reported if he left the house and was seen on the street.[4] He knew the outcome of his condition. He had read Norbert's letters and watched as they became shorter, more infrequent, and less optimistic. He knew that Norbert reported that his bumps were improving and that he held out hope for a cure that never came. He knew from his mother and father, if not personally,[5] the abject conditions of the hospital despite the compassion of the Daughters of Charity and, after 1921, the discipline of the military doctors in charge.[6] He had heard whispers in New Iberia and Lafayette, rumors about the reason for Norbert's disappearance. He knew about his brother's broken engagement. Leprosy and speculation about it had been conversation among the men at work at the drug company and Edmond had walked the streets of New Iberia, recognizing others with markings as damning as his own.

During the year-and-a-half that he spent confined to his home, Edmond was visited regularly by Dr. Sabatier, who demonstrated no fear of his patient, even sitting on Edmond's bed while scratching his own prickly summer heat. In this time, perhaps aided by Dr. Sabatier, Edmond tried to put his affairs in order. He was thirty-two, a young man now unable to provide for his twenty-six-year-old wife and two young children. Compensation from the government was slow in coming. Despite numerous letters to the Veterans Bureau, he never did receive the full military compensation he felt he deserved. Confined to his room, he could do little or nothing for his family. His situation was, in Arthur Frank's paradigm, "in chaos." It was at the opposite end of the continuum from the control which had been his for much of his life. His life now lacked words, for "chaos is what can never be told; it is the hole in the telling" (100–102 passim). Anger and depression must have haunted him. The discipline, determination, and work ethic that had impelled him in the past now failed and taunted him. Even the letters from Norbert had slowed and his earlier optimism had waned. Edmond could only imagine the fate that awaited him. He and Claire wrestled with their future: her fear for herself and their children, the futility of remaining homebound forever, the slim chance of remission, and the remote possibility that treatment in Carville might affect a cure or bring insight for them and for others with the disease. Edmond's time at home must have been lonely and painful, but I believe it was also fruitful, for it allowed him time to reflect on Norbert's fate, consider the life he would live in Carville, the value he could bring to that life, and the measures he could take to bring meaning to the lives of the patient community. At home, a prisoner in his own room, he began to consider options for his life in Carville and to find the freedom to voluntarily enter the United States Public Health Services Hospital #66.

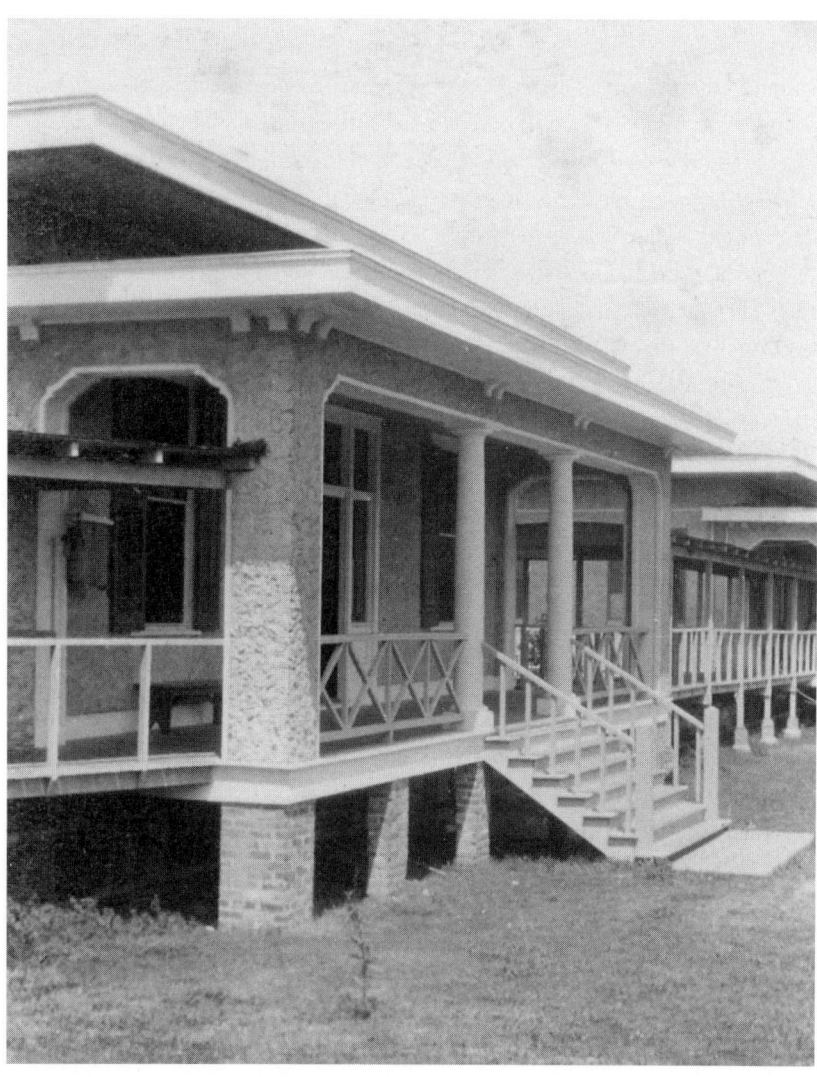

Men's Cottage, 1922–1938. Both Norbert and Edmond presumably lived in cottages such as this. (National Leprosarium. Photographer unknown. History of Carville, Vol. 1. Prints and Photographs Collection, National Hansen's Disease Programs Museum, Carville, LA. No. 47.)

CHAPTER 4

In Leprosy's Shadow: Life in Carville

"From the very beginning he became one of the outstanding leaders of our community"

1932 eulogy to Gabe Michael, *Sixty Six Star*

On September 11, 1924, one year and four months after Edmond had been confined to his home, incapacitated by leprosy, Dr. George Sabatier wrote to Dr. W. F. Carstens, Iberia Parish Health Officer and Edmond's personal friend, "Patient isolated, Healthy environment, but anxious to enter Leprosarium for treatment" (Edmond G. Landry, medical records). Less than a month later, on October 3, Dr. Carstens received word from Dr. Oscar Dowling, Louisiana State Board of Health President, to have "Mr. E. G. Landry *'leper'* [italics mine] 33, male, married sent forward" (Edmond G. Landry, medical records). Dr. Dowling also indicated that if Edmond were willing to go to Carville on his own there would be no need of interdiction, although he or his family would be expected to pay for his transportation. Dr. Dowling ended his letter, "Everything is now in readiness for his admission when he can be delivered at Carville" (Edmond G. Landry, medical records).

The die was cast; rules for disinfecting his home were issued, and on October 10, Edmond's twenty-seven-year-old wife, Claire, and her mother stood watching as he prepared to leave for the United States Public Health Services Hospital #66 in Carville for treatment of leprosy. Claire held her smiling three-year-old son, tow-headed Booz. Teenie, five, a strained smile on her face, hung close to her grandmother. Edmond kissed them all, told them he loved them, and left with his father, Terville, and his uncle, Henry. En route to the hospital, Edmond's luggage fell off of the car and the three men were forced to retrace their route to find the few possessions that Edmond had taken with him for the longest journey of his life.

The men traveled almost 170 miles on the same rough narrow roads that they had taken for four years in their visits to Norbert (who had died in Carville only eight months earlier despite his faithful regimen of prayer, medicine, and attention to his personal hygiene). They knew from experience Edmond's fate: the loss of citizenship privileges; no access to a telephone; and incarceration in a lonely hospital. They knew some of the patients and realized that the institution was filled with unwilling men, women, and children who were treated as outcasts, pitied and feared for their condition, or praised for their courage, but rarely viewed by outsiders as individual human beings with choice and dignity. Terville, Henry, and Edmond knew that leprosy was incurable but not terminal. They recalled that the federal hospital was run with military discipline that was challenged by the despondency and lethargy of patients who had little incentive to attend to their medical or personal needs. They knew of the unsanitary living conditions, and Edmond soon learned that the food was "no count." He was well aware of the requests Norbert had made for shaving soap, stationery, stamps, cigars, and a pocketknife, without which he felt lost. Edmond left for Carville with his eyes wide open, determined to make the best of his incarceration, and motivated to learn as much as he could about his condition.

My grandfather's entrance through the heavy iron gates of the hospital marked a new but unwanted phase of his life. His journey had been voluntary, but the reality was that his arrival marked incarceration, and only a documented cure would allow him a permanent and legitimate release from the hospital. Within minutes of his arrival, his fate confronted him as he saw the crippled limbs, blind eyes, and distorted faces of his fellow patients, silently daring Edmond to look at them.[1] They were the men, women, and children with whom he would spend the rest of his life. He may have come with good intentions to work for the benefit of himself and others, but on October 10, 1924, he was one among many whom society had cast aside.

He had a determination to be actively involved in the Carville community, but when he arrived at the hospital he was first treated as a passive patient, subjected to multiple examinations. His medical records confirmed his status as a patient. There are accounts of his medical history, dental records, temperature charts, and treatments. We learn his Carville alias,

Gabe Michael,[2] and his hospital number, 300. His records indicate that he was admitted to the hospital on October 10, 1924; that he needed a tooth extraction; had ingrown toenails on the big toe of each foot; that his feet were very painful; and that the muscles in both hands were weak. He was vaccinated with the smallpox virus and began the limited treatments for leprosy that were current at the time. He took chaulmoogra oil, until the 1940s the primary medication prescribed for leprosy. The drug was taken by injection, leaving patients with abscesses on their buttocks, or given orally, causing stomach distress. Daily hydrotherapy for his hands and feet was effective but slow. Edmond started treatment on his hands and feet in October, but it was not until December that a note was made, "hands, feet improved," and in February a notation said, "Hands and feet feeling very much better" (Edmond G. Landry, 1924–25 medical records).

In the collection of material on my grandfather, the only information available from October 1924 to February 1925 is the plethora of medical reports recording his condition and treatment. There are no letters indicating his activities or his inner struggles and no way to know the demons that assailed him. He had known since 1922 that leprosy was his fate, but in that time he still had some of the comforts of an ordinary life. Even isolated in his room in New Iberia, he experienced the hum of his household, the occasional guarded visits from his children, the comforts of a clean, well tended home, and the aromas from the kitchen: rich tomato gravies, green onions, and cakes and pies baking in the oven.

None of that existed in Carville, a place of loud raucous noise, vulgarity, little privacy, "no count food," and patients waiting in lines for meals, medication, bathroom facilities, and visits with the doctor. In the latter situation, patients would wait to see their doctors in an open room roped off from the medical office, leaving them with little occasion for private consultation. I once asked Mary Ruth, "How did you talk privately to the doctors?" She answered, "Oh, we stopped them in the halls." Bedrooms were regularly inspected, but this did not seem to insure their cleanliness or that of the common bathrooms, which included showers, toilet facilities, and a hopper that from the odor must have been used for more than washing. Armed guards patrolled the fenced-in grounds. Religious rituals, weekly movies, ball games, cards and gambling, a tennis court, and a nine-hole golf course offered some distraction to ease the deadly lethargy of the place. There were occasional dances and Mardi Gras celebrations that later included floats, doubloons, and a reigning king and queen.[3] Some patients developed an entrepreneurial spirit, using their skills to cater to the needs of the inmates and make a few dollars for themselves. Others used their skills to dupe patients and fill their own coffers. Despite all the activity, the institution was not home.

Added to the lethargy of the place were the constant reminders to the patients of their fate. In the 1920s, many walked haltingly or moved about on bicycles or wheelchairs on the covered boardwalks that connected the various wooden cottages. Their faces and extremities, often deformed by leprosy and sometimes wrapped in bandages, kept them all aware of the ravages of the disease and their condition as unwilling inmates in an unwelcoming environment. Even the huge sheltering oak trees, the proximity to the Mississippi River, and the lush "country club like surroundings"[4] gave little solace to those incarcerated there.

Edmond arrived in early October and anticipated in quick succession his thirty-third birthday on October 26, Thanksgiving, and Christmas. The holidays were celebrated in Carville with special meals, small gifts and prizes, and religious services, but none of that compared with the ongoing excitement of a home decorated for special occasions, a table covered with favorite food and drinks shared with family. Carville lacked the bright fall chrysanthemums in crystal bowls for Edmond's birthday or the deep green and red holly gracing tables and mantels for Christmas. Edmond longed for the succulent roast pork and turkey, stuffed with a savory bread dressing at Christmas, creations prepared by Claire with contributions from her in-laws' farm. There were no pecans, heady bourbon laced fruitcake, or cherry bounce. He imagined the magic and excitement of his children, left to celebrate Christmas without him. Despondency was heavy in this land of the living dead even as Edmond sought consolation in letters from home, prayer, the rituals of his Catholic religion, and his faith in God.

There are no existing letters from my grandfather to my grandmother or his family during his first eight months in Carville, although his first letters in 1925 seem to indicate that he had corresponded with the family. Maybe he wrote infrequently given that he got the blues whenever he sat down to write; maybe the letters were searing with despair and were thus read and destroyed; perhaps the family, still grieving Norbert's death, was not ready to accept Edmond's incarceration; or perhaps letters were written to Claire and she shared them with her in-laws and then destroyed them.[5]

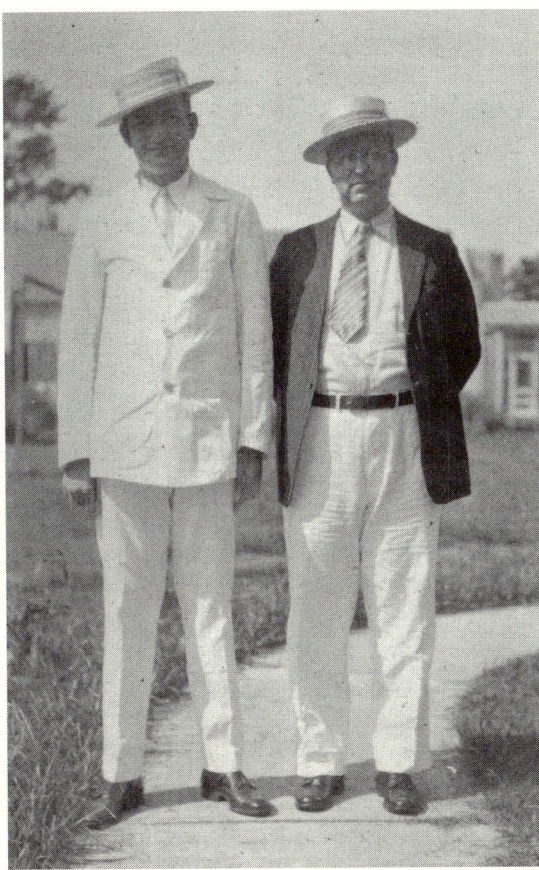

Edmond (right) and an un-
identified man at Carville.
In his letters my grandfather
spoke about Skipper, Eddie,
and Val, any one of whom
could be in this picture that
shows them "all dressed up
with perhaps no place to
go." (Date unknown; family
photo; used with permission.)

Although there are no known remaining letters to his family during
1924, Edmond was active in his early months in Carville. He quickly set
about making a life for himself in the colony separate from his family life.
He directed his family to write to him so that he received their letters on
Fridays and could answer them right away. Perhaps early on he also acquired a private cottage like so many of those cobbled together by other
patients.[6] This gave him time, space, and quiet away from the disorderly and
sometimes noisy activity in the hospital's apartments. The first letter in his
records indicates that by February 1925, Edmond was the secretary and treasurer of the "What Cheer Club," a patient organization begun by my grandfather to administer funds from the patient canteen, which he also founded
and managed without a salary. Stanley Stein, author and a Carville patient,
wrote in his memoir *Alone No Longer* that the canteen afforded patients the

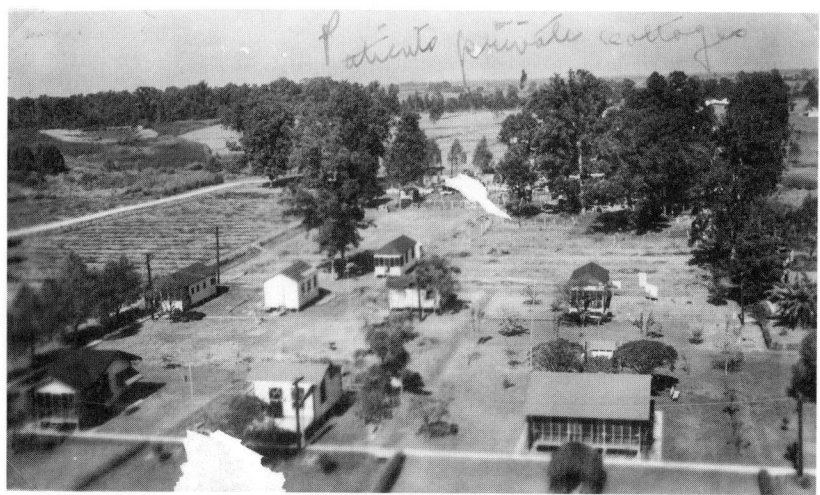

An aerial view of the private cottages in Carville. Edmond at some point acquired a private cottage, which he offered for some of the Carville parties. (Private Patients' Cottages, 1940s[?]. National Leprosarium. History of Carville, Vol. 2. Prints and Photographs Collection, National Hansen's Disease Programs Museum; Carville, LA. No. 39.)

opportunity to buy items not ordinarily available to them (59).[7] The money from the canteen was then used to aid the blind and indigent patients.[8]

Letters from my grandfather between 1925 and his death in Carville in 1932 attest to his keen attention to the needs of others. He read and wrote letters for those who were unable to do so on their own. He visited the sick and dying when others had given up on them. He shared his food and money with the needy. In 1928, when he was at his lowest, he nonetheless offered himself as a subject for examination at a medical conference in New Orleans.[9]

Throughout his time in Carville, Edmond's effort to work for the good of the patient community took varying forms. Stanley Stein noted that in 1931 Gabe Michael, "in an effort to lift the patient body out of its deadly lethargy . . . had organized a minstrel show in which he was going to be the interlocutor" (53). My grandfather's fidelity to the Carville community was also evident in his participation with the group of veterans in Carville who met in June 1931 with Sam Jones, then Louisiana Commander of the American Legion and later governor of Louisiana. It was a meeting that Stein described as "the day of our breakthrough" (117). The meeting was a protest by those who had served their country in war and were now incarcerated patients cast aside by their families and their government. Many were unable to receive the compensation due them; all felt their isolation and their status as castaways, but they still met to demand their rights. Stein quotes Jones extensively in relation to the visit. Jones notes that the patients were "men of good minds, many well educated yet mentally haywire because they were convinced they were pariahs. . . . One chap said, 'Mr. Jones, we're the bottom. You won't find anybody lower than we are'" (119). This group presented their needs: "a decent infirmary building, a recreation hall to replace the filthy canteen, more contact with the world outside, if only with outside baseball teams to play on the Carville diamond" (118). The meeting gave Carville residents a legitimacy and dignity they had previously not experienced, planted the seed for a Carville post of the American Legion, and initiated a longstanding and still existing relationship between the American Legion and Hansen's disease patients. The requests for facilities were slow in coming, but before my grandfather died in 1932 he wrote that work had begun on the new infirmary. When Edmond's sister, Amelie, arrived in 1934, she noted that the family would not recognize the place because of the changes.

My grandfather's interests in Carville were not only political. Shortly after Stanley Stein arrived as a patient in Carville in 1931, he began an in-house newspaper, the *Sixty Six Star*, which became the forerunner of the international magazine *The Star*, whose mission statement was, "Radiating the light of truth on Hansen's Disease." Early issues of the paper connected patients with one another and shared news, gossip, and commentary from the patient community. According to the paper, my grandfather was one of the first to purchase a subscription to the paper and he conducted readings of the *Sixty Six Star* on Friday evenings at 5:30 *prompt* for those who were unable to read the paper themselves. On occasion, he offered his assistance to the patient news staff, also disabled by leprosy. He helped, despite his own weak and numb hands, to type copy on a heavy old manual typewriter.

He was also the subject of some of the news in the paper, which recorded visits to Gabe Michael by his wife and family. On several occasions, he entertained friends at his cottage and offered his home for parties hosted by others. Two accounts in particular attest to the cheerfulness of those events. The August 8, 1931, issue reports that "a group of Kona Singh's [sic] gathered at Gabe Michael's cottage on Monday evening and enjoyed a delicious chicken dinner 'with all the trimmings.' Mr. Singh who will be leaving the Colony soon having received his discharge was the recipient of many hearty good wishes for his future welfare." In the July 23, 1932, issue there is a report of another party with even more festivity. "One of the gayest events of the season was held last Sunday evening at Gabe's cottage as a farewell to Miss Olga. The affair started off with a delicious dinner under the supervision of George Alexis [who 'in pre-Carville days' had been a chef at a swanky hotel in the East" (Stein, 167)]. This was followed by dancing during which refreshments were served. The party waxed merry until midnite and then after the guests had departed, the Glee Club Boys who furnished the music decided to further express their good wishes by serenading Olga neath her window[.]"

Gabe generously offered his cottage for entertainment, but he was still perceived as straight laced, as the June 13, 1931, Colony Capers in the *Sixty Six Star* notes, "Swallow this one: Gabe seen reading sensational dime novels! 'Nick Carter' or the 'Great Train Robbery'—no foolin'!" He may have seemed stern but he also had a wry sense of humor when he wanted to make a point. In an October 1931 issue of the paper, he wrote, "Early to bed and early to rise, and in house 41 there's a lot of loud guys."

While my grandfather related to and cared for others, his files indicate that he also took agency for himself in a time before such self-determination was considered appropriate by the medical community.[10] He wrote more than once to the Veterans Bureau attempting to receive the full benefits that he felt were due him and his family. At times he requested that some of his treatments be stopped and he read widely about his condition.[11] On one occasion, he wrote a medical professor in Cuba requesting information on choroiditys in leprosy patients. Although his letter and money were returned through Dr. Denney, he had clearly taken responsibility for his condition. His concern for his children was evident from the gifts that he sent them. "Whatever we needed, he sent us," is the way my mother recalls his generosity. "Mamma must have told him what we needed and he got it for us." She remembers in particular a radio console and a set of the *Encyclopedia Britannica* with the cabinet to hold the books. He grieved over the absence of and silence about his daughter and son, yet maintained his isolation in Carville lest they be further exposed to leprosy.

My grandfather entered into the life of Carville and involved himself in his own treatment, but he was no saint. He had his demons. He could be demanding of himself and others, angry and impatient with bureaucracy as he perceived it and with his unjust incarceration in Carville. He was unfaithful to his wife and separated himself from the rituals of the Church to which he had been devoted. He struggled with the desire to abscond or to end his life, but it was this very darkness that gives credence to his life.

In his eight years and two months in Carville, Edmond returned home only twice, both times accompanied by armed and uniformed guards.[12] To this day, his daughter neither forgives nor fully understands the experience of seeing her father standing along side two armed men in military hats and holsters. When I asked her what she thought about the armed guards. she said, "I don't know maybe we [Booz and I] thought he was in prison." My grandfather never left Carville permanently and he never became the successful businessman or banker he may have aspired to be, but his life was one of significance and witness for himself, the Carville community, and his family. In his life in New Iberia, he had been recognized by Dr. Carstens, his personal friend, as a "mighty good citizen, an exemplary father and husband" who was "valued highly by our entire community" (Carstens to Denney, October 8, 1924, Edmond Landry medical records), and Dr. Denney called him "one of our few really good citizens" (Denney to Dr. L. H. Webb, October 19, 1925, Edmond G. Landry medical records). After my grandfather's death, Dr. F. A. Johansen, the attending physician, wrote to my grandmother that he "died honored and respected by all of us" (letter to Mrs. Claire G. Landry, December 7, 1932, collection). Not only the medical and religious staff wrote respectfully of him, but the patient population who knew him at his best and at his lowest also expressed their admiration in a eulogy in the *Sixty Six Star*. They acknowledged: [with] "Gabe Michael— . . . a new force came into being which was to effect profoundly not alone the life of the community as a whole, but the lives of many of the individuals composing it as well. . . . [And in death his name] was scratched from the hospital roster, but the force which it represented continues alive and potent."

Now years after his death he has also become a witness for me and his other descendants who continue to plumb the meaning of his life and who have tried to discover, represent, and honor the dignity of this man we call our grandfather.

Carville, La
June 5, 1925.

Dear Folks:—

Guess you all were ___ ___ last Sunday as I don't think the mail went out until Monday morning. You all no doubt realized after that it was due to the holiday.

Received Amelie's letter to-day and was glad to hear from her— I prefer to receive your letters on Friday so I can answer them right away instead of the following Friday when I received them on Saturday or Sunday.

It certain is too bad about Lawrence's wife and

Edmond's first extant letter to his family was written in June 1925. It is his longest to his folks and sets some of the themes of his life in Carville. In this first page he separates his family life and his Carville life. (Landry Letters from Carville; used with permission.)

CHAPTER 5

Edmond's Letters from Carville

Letters can never adequately reveal the anguish of a life lived separated from family, but they are courageous attempts at doing just that. While they may not ever fully express the passion of the heart, they are still an immediate and direct contact with loved ones. When Edmond sat down in Carville to write to his family, he was closeted in his cell-like bedroom, which contained a bed, a desk, books, a typewriter, and a small armoire or closet for his few possessions. The most recent framed picture of his wife and two children hung on the wall, as did a calendar that haunted with its meaningless count of days. His hands were crippled and numbed by leprosy, and he got the blues whenever he wrote, but he wrote, nonetheless, to his wife and family. His most frequent signature to his family was "As ever, Edmond," as though in his single-minded effort to overcome the grief, anger, and lethargy that made letter writing so painful, he asserted his identity. He was Edmond: son, brother, husband, father, ever the same no matter the condition of his skin and the stigmatization to his person.

I have learned to know him as my grandfather and as Edmond, but my knowledge of him is mediated by years, by my mother's few memories, by changing attitudes toward Hansen's disease, and by his old letters. When he wrote what are now the fading, yellowed remnants of his correspondence, he was writing with an immediacy that only letters could give. He had no access to a phone; visits from his wife and family were infrequent and non-existent from his kids. His two or three brief visits home were less than satisfactory. Only in his correspondence could he record his life, and even then he sifted his narratives and tailored the voice he used in each of the three sets of letters contained here. The letters to his folks, pages 48–83, are the letters of a son trying to relate the more ordinary aspects of his life to those he loved. No doubt he omitted many of the bleaker descriptions of his internment lest his family, too, be caught in the darkness of leprosy. To his wife, he wrote letters which were sometimes shared with his parents and read, carefully edited, to his children. The two remaining letters to his wife, pages 84–123, reveal more forcefully his anger, loneliness, and desperation than does the collection to his folks.

His third set of letters, pages 125–39, written to hospital and government officials, are more official and businesslike, and are signed Gabe Michael or Edmond G. Landry, depending on the circumstances. They were brief, succinct, sometimes abrupt and demanding but all were indicative of his sense of autonomy.

Dear Folks—As Ever Edmond

> *"This surely is a 'lepers' place."*
> Edmond to Family, January 11, 1926

....

Carville, La.
June 5, 1925

Dear Folks,

Guess you all were [surprised] last Sunday as I don't think the mail went out until Monday morning. You all no doubt realized after that it was due to the holiday.

Received Amelie's letter today and was glad to hear from her. I prefer to receive your letters on Friday so I can answer them right away instead of the following Friday when I receive them on Saturday or Sunday.

It certainly is too bad about Lawrence's wife and leaving such a young baby.

I received the box of peaches yesterday and it is useless for me to say that they were enjoyed. They are not so big but they are delicious. I gave a few out but kept most for myself as they are well preserved. Many thanks for same.

Received Marie's letter last Saturday and was glad to hear from her.

Glad to hear that Ulysses' father is improving.

Sorry to hear of Judge Simon's illness and Mr. Blanchette's death. All these high livers generally kickoff suddenly.

Wish I could have been there to enjoy some of Uncle Henry's crawfish. We never get any here. We had crabs (Gumbo) for supper but they were not fresh enough so they lack the flavor.

Mrs. W. went home on some business last Sunday and came back last night. I have not heard for what reason but it is not on account of sickness.

I saw Sr. R[egina] to nite after services and she told me to thank you all for the peaches which she received today for her and to say that they were very much appreciated. I had gone to the hospital to see Alex who is very low and his friends, mostly all, went back on him and he takes it hard to be without visitors. I generally call on him every day but don't think that I will have many more visits to pay him.

The employees (outside) will play another game on our diamond tomorrow again. They played a pretty good game last Saturday and the losing side wants their revenge.

Just got a radio report of some fight and you would think the fight was right in here with all the excitement.

I am still feeling fine and my feet are giving me very little trouble. The Rays have improved my legs wonderfully.

Saturday Morning

Last night I ran out of news and went to bed leaving this open in case that I would think of anything else.

Had hard luck with my white pants. The first time I had them washed the pair was scorched. I had given them to a new man to wash so as to help him out as he had no money. It is not scorched very badly and he claims he can remove it the next time he washes them.

We have very heavy fog here this morning. You can't see the houses from one side to the other.

Well I must clean my monkey cage for inspection so will have to close.

Love and kisses to all

As ever

Edmond

This June letter is the first extant one from Edmond to his family and the longest to his mother and father. It serves as prologue to the remaining letters to his folks. Here he sets the parameters of his life in Carville, wanting to receive letters from home on Fridays so that he could answer them right away. He seems to be setting a clear distinction between his life in Carville as a patient and his lost family life in New Iberia. Weekdays were for Carville business and medicine, but weekends, often slower and lonelier, allowed time for correspondence and perhaps for visitors.

He lives in a "monkey cage" that is inspected weekly. The term is apt, for patients participated in various treatments for leprosy which could have made them feel like lab monkeys, and at times they were viewed by outsiders as subjects of curiosity much like monkeys in a cage. On one occasion in the 1920s, a patient was on trial in Baton Rouge. The case was probably highly publicized and attracted the attention of curious onlookers. One account told of a woman with her son in tow asking a group of strangers on the street if they were here to see "them." I can only imagine her dismay when the strangers boarded a bus clearly labeled "Lepers Home" and left for Carville.

This letter sets other themes as well. My grandfather determinedly uses his baptismal name, Edmond, with his family, rather than his Carville name, Gabe Michael. His appreciation of letters from home and his concern for those who are ill keep him connected to family, as does the food he receives from them. The food bridges the expanse between home and hospital as he mentions frequently sharing his treats with others. He shares not only his food but himself as he maintains a concern for the sick in Carville, visiting them when they seem to have been forgotten by others.

His benign comment about his white pants being scorched amuses me. He had been frugal at school and in the army and here he is unconcerned that his good pants might have been ruined. He had given them to a patient who did laundry "to help him out," and he was unconcerned about the possible loss.

October 2, 1925

Dear Folks,

I received Marie's letter last Monday and as usual was glad to hear from her.

I am glad to say that we are not bothered with mosquitoes. We have been having rain nearly every day and some pretty strong blows also.

Was very sorry to hear of Amelie being under the weather but hope she is alright by now.

With all the rains falling it seems as though the wells should start filling up instead of staying dry.

We had crab gumbo for supper but it was no count as usual. They don't know how to make it.

It will be a good thing if they run a double track to Lafayette. They are always better than single tracks.

That Frenchman from Milton died this evening at 5:30 so I just heard. They will have a hard time finding his people as I wrote for him 3 weeks ago and never got any answer. He was in very bad shape when he came.

We have prayers every day this month. The Catholic part of my gang surely hates the idea but if they miss prayers they have to miss a show so they are very punctual.

I am feeling alright except that the oil [chaulmoogra] made me sick this afternoon but it has passed tonight.

Guess Claire told you all about the samples of pecans so don't forget them. A man from California wants to have some mailed to his home if he likes them.

I want to go to bed early and catch up my sleep as I got up early to go to church this morning. I have to write another letter before going to bed for a crippled patient.

Love and kisses to all
As ever
Edmond

"Was sorry to hear of Amelie." Amelie was eighteen at this time and had shown signs of leprosy at least as early as 1923. This illness may have been connected with the disease. Dr. Sabatier had a progressive view of the disease and did not automatically report a patient who showed signs of leprosy.

"*That Frenchman . . .*" Edmond's simple lines tell a stark story. Patients were frequently abandoned by their families once they entered the hospital. As in this case, they were often in bad shape when they came because they hid as long as they could before seeking what little treatment Carville offered.

"*I wrote for him . . .*" Both in the army and in Carville, Edmond recounts writing for some of the men. My grandfather was bilingual, writing and speaking both French and English. This letter may have been in French since he specifically mentions that the man is a Frenchman.

"*We have prayers . . .*" Although by 1925, the Daughters of Charity were no longer in charge of the hospital there was a Catholic chaplain and chapel on the grounds. Novenas, rosaries, and other devotions were available, but not obligatory, to the Catholic population in the Carville hospital. This comment about having to attend prayers or not being able to attend the weekly shows is confusing. Edmond at some point was in charge of the young male patients. I presume he made the attendance at prayers mandatory for his young charges if they wanted to attend the movies shown weekly at the hospital.

Carville, La.
Jan. 11, 1926

Dear Folks:—

I received mamma and Amelie's letters and was very glad to hear from them both. I also received the prayer bead that Mr. G. sent me and appreciate his thoughtfulness very much. It is a very rare souvenir. Thank him very kindly for same when you see him, for me.

No doubt you all have been wondering why I did not write. Well it is just that I had to, as I did not want to answer mamma's letter for I do not know how to. I am sorry she was brought in but understand and appreciate her feeling and her interest in my behalf. The only thing I can say is that anyone here feels as I do and anyone who knows what I know and told Claire and she knows to be facts feels as I do. I am less of a "leper" to-day than I've been since after that bad case of flue. The only trouble is that everybody knows it now and no one knew it then. I could say lots more but you all can't help me so it is useless for me to burden you all with my troubles. I am just trying

to adjust myself to this place for it is truly a "lepers" place. Lots go
but lots come back God only knows why. They won't say but I think
I know why.
    I am well as can be and send love to all.

As ever
Edmond

"*No doubt you all have been wondering . . .*" By 1926, Edmond and Claire
were having trouble. He longed for his wife and knew that there was little
risk of her contracting leprosy, but she was torn between her love for him
and her fear for their children. Edmond's father, Terville, visited his grandchildren and daughter-in-law when he came into town from the Landry
home on Spanish Lake. Perhaps Claire had confided in him and shared letters she had received from Edmond. Claire was only twenty-eight at this
time and maybe overwhelmed by her life.

"*Lots go but lots come back. . . . They won't say but I think I know why.*"
Edmond does not explain his remark, but in the 1920s public fear and ignorance of leprosy were rampant and left many people stigmatized both in
and out of Carville. The treatment of leprosy patients outside of the hospital may have forced some to return to Carville. In a long letter to Claire
(pages 92–123), Edmond reports that patients left the hospital only to be
returned there by family who had purported to want them home. In her
books *Miracle at Carville* and *No One Must Ever Know*, Betty Martin writes
of the challenge of trying to live anonymously on the outside.

Even in the 1940s and '50s, Carville residents still struggled with being
identified as patients from the hospital. Mary Ruth, a longtime friend who
died in 2004, tells of a trip that she, her husband Daryl, and other patients
took to New Orleans, perhaps escaping through the hole in the fence. They
spent a few hours at a well-known bar in a downtown New Orleans hotel,
hoping to remain anonymous, lost in the crowd; instead, they were greet-
ed across the bar by a woman familiar with Carville. She waved and cried
loudly, "How are things in Carville?" The greeting was innocent on the
friend's part but disconcerting to the Carville patients who knew only too
well the fear their presence could evoke. On another occasion Mary, Daryl,
and others attended an LSU football game in Tiger Stadium. As they set-
tled into the bleachers they looked up to see doctors from the hospital also

ready to enjoy the game. Mary laughingly recalled the way the patients scurried to find seats farther away from the scrutiny of the doctors. Their LSU trip was still "breaking the Carville laws," but neither doctors nor patients acknowledged the encounter. Staying in Carville was not pleasant, but trips out, even for a few hours, had risks.

Carville, La.
Jan. 18, 1926

Dear Folks,
I received Marie's letter last Saturday and was glad to hear from her.
I put off writing Friday to Sunday and Sunday I did not feel like writing so put it off again to Monday night but we had Club business to come up and I had to make reports on absconders so I could not get to it. I am dropping you all a few lines so you all will not be worried.
I received the box yesterday and appreciate same very much.
Hope the new tenant proves to be as good as you all think.
Outside of my ear still hurting and a head and chest cold I am doing well.

Lots of love to all
As ever
Edmond

[March or April 1926. This undated fragment mentions Father Keenan who died on March 22, 1926.]

Father Keenan, the priest who used to be here a few years ago, died Friday a week ago with the flue Some of the Sisters went to his funeral. It might have been on the papers but I did not see anything about it. Of course it is very seldom I read any papers.
There are all kinds of petitions going around here now. Some wants to put the sisters and the priest out others are petitioning to have Dr. W. fired but I tell them they are all losing their time, nothing will be done.

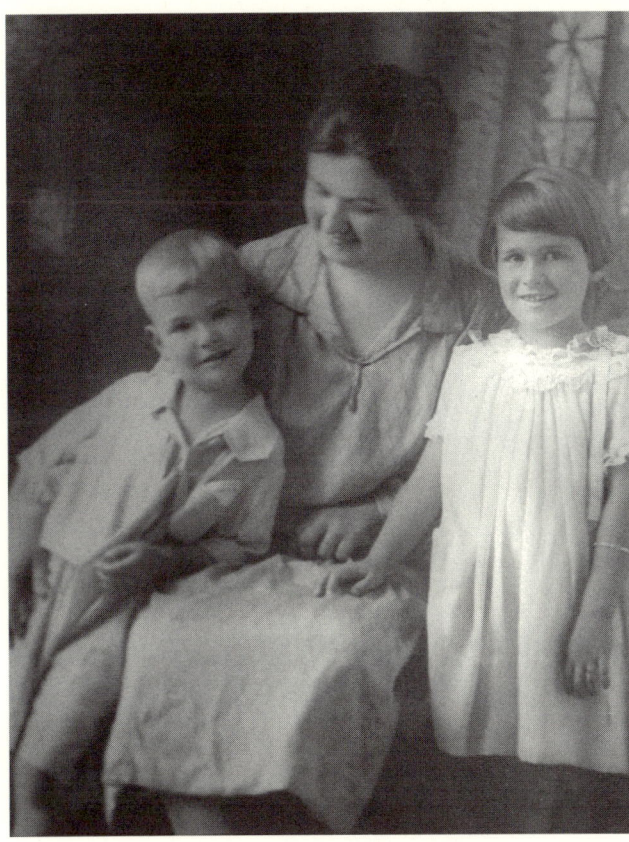

Claire (29) with Booz (5) and Teenie (7) in a photo for Edmond's thirty-fifth birthday (October 1926). (Family collection; used with permission.)

We are expecting the Stanacola Band here for a concert to-morrow. They will also put on a boxing match.

This will be all for this time.

Lots of love to all
As ever
Edmond

"There are all kinds of petitions going around here now." Even during the days when Carville was a state run institution, patients were politically active, as noted by Michelle T. Moran in her work *Colonizing Leprosy: Imperialism and the Politics of Public Health in the United States*, so it is not surprising that disgruntled, incarcerated patients would demand their rights. Although Edmond, realistically or cynically, held out little hope

of success in this incident, on several occasions patients did have their voices heard. In 1931, Edmond was part of a group of veterans who won the support of Sam Jones and the American Legion forging a relationship that has lasted until today. Mary Ruth recalled that in 1939 the Patients' Federation was successful in having a Medical Officer in Charge assigned elsewhere. In the 1950s, the Patients' Federation again lobbied for their demands to be met, and in the 1990s, it was the patients and their political network that kept the hospital open even after other Public Health Hospitals had been shut down. Although the United States Public Health Hospital was ultimately closed, patient activism helped to ensure that aging patients unable or unwilling to leave would be cared for, and medical treatment for life, as well as monetary compensation, was available to those who chose to leave.

"We are expecting the Stanacola Band . . ." Various groups from the surrounding areas would come to Carville to entertain in the pavilion or later in the auditorium. Ball teams, too, would visit to compete against the patients on their home diamond.

Carville, La
May 7, 1926

Dear Folks,

I am busy and did not expect to write but as Sunday is Mother's Day, it would not be right to let mamma and of course all of you, without a letter

Skipper is sick and I am looking after his work and mine with Carlos helping me but he is new on the job and is not very much help just now.

Everything that you all brought on both trips was delicious. You should have seen the two kids we had with us mop up on mutton.

There is nothing new around here and I am feeling the same.

With love to all
As ever
Edmond

Hope they made the trip in good time and without any trouble.

"*Skipper and Carlos*" may have been my grandfather's assistants in the canteen since the business needed staff to maintain the shelves, update inventory, service the customers, and cash payroll checks.

Carville, La.
Nov. 5, 1926

Dear Folks:—
    I received Mamma's letter last Saturday and was very glad to hear from her.
    I appreciated very much the money sent as birthday remembrance [Edmond's birthday was October 26]. I will get me a shirt later on with it. I also received the candies. Many thanks for all.
    Yes my actions were funny looking and I don't blame you all for not understanding and I don't want any one to understand. The fact is that I don't hardly understand myself. But nevertheless I could not do what I wanted and I did not mention anything about it in my other letter because I did not know whether Claire had told you all or not and if she had not told, it was no use for me to bring it up. I first told her to tell you all but thought that on the second part of the letter I had said, 'never mind saying anything to the folks' but I must have overlooked it. You all need not worry about me here or outside—good or bad weather—as I told Claire—'Hotel takes anyone's money and not ones blood tests and there are lots of doctors who will treat even a "leper."' Thank God for that.
    Everything here is still the same and I am doing fairly well.

Lots of love to all,
As ever
Edmond

"*I will get me a shirt . . .*" Some clothes were provided to patients, but they also had access to mail order catalogs, and Mary Ruth, who came to Carville in 1939, recalls choosing clothes from racks that were set up in the yard near the infirmary. As Mary Ruth recalled these transactions, the clothes were on racks on one side of the hedge that separated the patient side from the staff side of the institution. Patients pointed to clothes that they wanted and someone brought the garments to them. It was not clear to me if these were the hospital-issued clothes or those brought in by a merchant. Mary also recalls that at the time, women's underpants were long unattractive pantaloons. She and her sister, Kitty, also a patient, requested better garments from their mother who sewed the garments for them.

"*Yes my actions were funny looking . . .*" This paragraph remains mysterious although it would seem that my grandfather was thinking of absconding from the hospital or legally seeking treatment on the outside. Earlier letters obliquely indicate Edmond's struggles, and a long letter, pages 93–123, written in June 1928, indicates that Edmond and Claire had long had difficulties after his entrance to Carville, and that he had at one time wished to return home, but his wife had refused. My cousin Paul remembers reading a letter, now missing, in which our grandfather threatened to take his children and move to Brazil. Perhaps the letter to Claire referred to here in 1926, is that missing correspondence. It certainly helps to give credence to the crisis that came to a head in 1928 and explains the remarks about hotels taking money not blood.

Carville, La.
Feb. 16, 1927

Dear Folks,

I received Amelie's letter and was glad to hear from her.

I received, also today, a box of candy and one cooked chicken. Both of which were enjoyed very much. I was very hungry to-nite. Eddie, Helen and I ate the whole chicken by ourselves except two sandwiches which we gave to a blind boy and a crippled one. Many thanks.

We have been very busy at the canteen. Inventory sale—inventory taking and now pricing it. When that is thru I have to audit the books and make out a semi-annual report. I'll be busy the balance of the month so would ask you all to wait until about the second Sunday in March to come to see me. As on the first of each month I render a monthly statement and collect about 75 accounts and also cash about $3000.00 worth of $15.00 and $40.00 checks.

Hope Albert will be able to get off. Hope also that he likes his job and is doing well, even tho he is away from home. I am and have to

*like it with all its disadvantages as much as I could and want to be
away from here.*

*Just copied, today the enclosed article from a paper. It's nice to
be a politician. Others here from the same state were sent out at once
and robbed of their property after they got here. You show it to Claire.*

Everything here is still the same.

*As ever
Edmond*

"*We have been very busy* . . ." My grandfather had founded the canteen
and for a time worked there without taking a salary.

"*Also cash about $3000.00 worth* . . ." Some patients received insurance
benefits and those who were able to helped with services at the hospital
and were paid a small remuneration. This may explain the checks that my
grandfather cashed at the canteen.

"*Hope Albert will be able to get off* . . ." Albert moved from New Iberia
sometime after he completed high school, worked for the telephone company as a lineman and married a woman from Opelousas. My cousin Paul
theorizes that he moved to escape the family disease and the stigma.

"*Just copied, today the enclosed article* . . ." My grandfather seems understandably bitter about the inequity in the treatment of patients diagnosed
with leprosy but his remarks also indicate the discrepancy in views about
the need for incarceration.

*Carville, La
Mar. 6, 1927*

*Dear Folks,
    Just a few lines to say that I am glad to hear that you all expect to
come next Sunday and hope the weather will be good.*

Will keep all the rest for when you all come.

I am feeling fine as can be expected.

*Love to all.
As ever
Edmond*

The Great Mississippi River flood in the spring of 1927 caused massive destruction along its banks, but my grandfather does not mention it in any letters to his folks. In an April letter to Claire, page 86, he does admit his fear and concern about the event and asks for her help if the levee were to break.

Carville, La.
Aug. 8, 1927

Dear Folks,

I received mamma's letter yesterday and was glad to hear from her. I know that it has been long since I wrote and I am to blame but there is always one thing or another that makes me put off from day to day.

Was to write Friday but we had a big excitement that afternoon and I could not. The excitement was indeed a sad one as one patient shot and killed another. Shot him nine times.

He was buried today. All kinds of red tape and humbug. They took the murderer out for safe keeping. Of course those kinds of news don't get in the papers. The officer keeps that out of the papers.

He owed me money so now I'll have to file claim against his insurance.

Two of my clerks have been sick and that has kept me closer on the job. They are both back today. Good thing for next week is stock taking.

I am sorry that mamma has been suffering with headaches again.

I rec'd several letters from Aunt A[drienne] which I never answered but God know[s] I like to hear from them and mean to write but what is there for me to tell them that they have not heard of through you all. And if I want to get a real good case of hard blue I just got to sit down to write a letter and as I said before that is also one reason for my not writing oftener and it makes me feel worse when I am reproached about not writing even though I deserve it.

Now I've tried to answer mamma's question about Easter Duties by not answering it hoping it would be understood that I had not made them without my saying so. Well the fact is that I have not and am very sorry but dear folks as bad as it is not to make them,

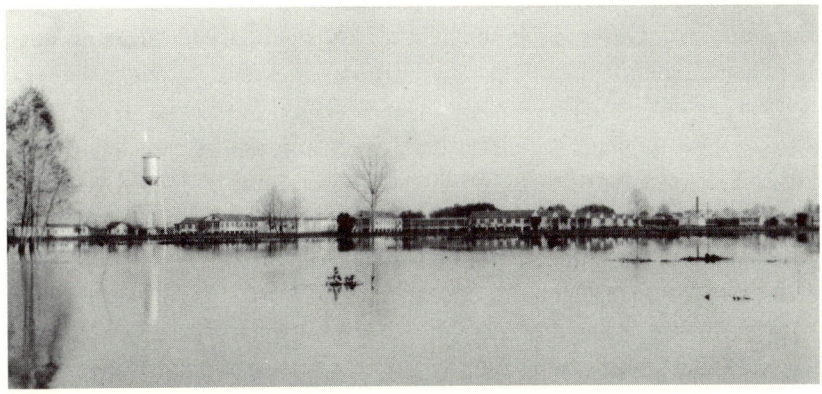

The Great Mississippi River Flood of 1927 impacted Carville but did not necessitate evacuation of the residents or staff. (1927 Flood, National Leprosarium, Carville, LA. Photographer unknown. History of Carville, Vol. 1. Prints and Photographs Collection, National Hansen's Disease Programs Museum, Carville, LA; No. 14.)

there are certain conditions in which I am that making them would be worse yet.

There are certain dispositions required to make a good communion and I can't meet them now. I can't ask the Lord for help. All I ask Him is for mercy and I have still Faith in Him in my way as bad as I may appear to be. I do all I can to help all those less fortunate than me and hope in Him for forgiveness in passing up Easter Duties instead of making a bad one.

"A tout paché miserecord."

John has taken another turn for the better and has improved much. Joe and Mrs. S. will leave in a few days.

I am still the same as when you all were here.

Lots of love to all
As ever
Edmond

"*We had a big excitement that afternoon . . .*" There is a strange dissonance in my grandfather's reaction to the murder. He is sad but also frustrated with the red tape of the institution and bothered that he will now have to file a claim against the man's insurance. This incident also invites speculation about the conflict facing Carville authorities. The shooter would not have been safe at the hospital but would not have been wanted in prison either.

"Now I've tried to answer mamma's question about Easter Duties . . ." Easter Duties refer to the obligation Catholics have to receive Holy Communion at least once a year during the Easter season (which lasts until Pentecost Sunday). To receive Communion, one has to be in a state of grace and free of mortal sin. Edmond indicates that he cannot fulfill this expectation. Nothing is ever said directly but it is possible that Edmond was living or had been living with a female patient in Carville and was not willing to relinquish this relationship. As he further indicates in this letter to his folks, he does good for those who need it and he relies solely on the mercy of God. For a man who had been faithful to his religion and taken comfort in its rituals, this total dependence on God without access to the rituals of religion is a profound act of faith.

1928—A YEAR OF CRISIS

My grandfather entered Carville in October 1924 and died there in December of 1932. 1928 was the middle of his incarceration. According to the letters he wrote during that year, it was a year fraught with sacrifice and pain. Some of the letters to his family are confusing and present him as distracted and searching for assistance. Correspondence with the Veterans Bureau indicates that he may have considered absconding or committing suicide (page 132), yet in a letter to Dr. Denney (page 134) during this same period he expresses his willingness to demonstrate his illness to a group of medical personnel in New Orleans. His letter to his wife Claire, composed during the early part of 1928 and mailed in June, gives the longest and clearest demonstration of his pain. In the midst of his anguish he also shows that he was assuming clear responsibility for his life.

Carville, Louisiana
February 24, 1928

Dear Folks:
    I received Amelie's letter and was glad to hear from her, as usual.

Many thanks for getting Edwin Broussard's address. Guess I'll have to write him, as it may be a long time before he gets back to New Iberia.

This week I wrote to Dr. Carstens and asked him to come to see me as I needed him to help me in something. Guess he will see papa about it. Of course if he can't come, I will take the matter up by mail but I would prefer to speak to him as one gets better understanding by talking than by correspondence

I've been busy to-day, as I change rooms. I moved from number 8 room to number 9, as it has a bigger locker. One never knows how much junk he has until he starts moving.

Outside of a few deaths and a few new patients things here are about the same. I am doing well outside of my cough and nerve-pain, but to-day they are both better especially the pains.

Lots of love to all
As ever,
Edmond

"*Edwin Broussard*" from New Iberia was a Louisiana senator at this time. It is possible that Edmond was writing a political letter to Broussard on his own behalf or that of another patient.

"*Dr. Walter Carstens*" was the Chief Health Officer for Iberia parish. There was a personal relationship between my grandfather and Dr. Carstens: he and his wife were neighbors of Edmond and Claire, and the doctor shared office space in the Estorge Drug Company where Edmond had worked. Dr. Carstens had written a letter on my grandfather's behalf when Edmond entered Carville. I do not know what help my grandfather wanted, but his correspondence in 1928 raises many questions. Could Dr. Carstens have helped him with a discharge? Would he have helped Edmond abscond? Did Edmond perhaps think that Dr. Carstens could alleviate Claire's fear of leprosy? I can only speculate, but certainly Edmond's correspondence in 1928 indicates a crisis in his life.

"*I've been busy to-day . . .* " My grandfather's letters in early 1928 seem contradictory and confusing, the actions of a man at a crossroads. He moves to a bigger room even as he might have been contemplating suicide or absconding.

Mar. 14, 1928

Dear Folks:—

I received Amelie's letter to-day and was glad to hear from you all.

I evidently forgot to tell you all about my having my checks mailed home. Well like any mail addressed there just forward same to me here.

We had a splendid trip to N.O. Several patients and I were taken down there to show different stages of this disease. No one not even the Doctors would believe that I had it, but when it is all said and done, in my good physical condition I am, by far, worse off than some in pretty bad shape here.

Sometime ago mamma said a patient could not get along outside. Well one went out 4½ [years] ago and staid out 3 years but got tired of having no close companion and came back 17 months ago and has had good tests ever since and will be discharged next month and he is in far worse shape than I [am] physically of course we can't say this to outsiders.

Glad to hear that Albert will possibly be transferred back home and hope mamma will have luck with her chickens.

My N.O. trip and lots I learned on it made me realize the injustice and uselessness of isolation more than ever but that is of no good to me except to make life more miserable to me.

One man was there from the outside scared of us, not knowing what he had—and he is here to-day one of us, expecting to be cured in 3 weeks.

Lots of love to all
As ever
Edmond

"*Having my checks mailed home.*" By itself, this comment sheds little light on Edmond's state of mind. However, the combination of this with an earlier letter to his family on February 24, 1928, a letter to the Veterans Bureau on February 22 (page 132), and one to Dr. Denney on February 28 or 29 (page 134) indicate a conflicted man. He has his checks sent home, perhaps so the family could get them if he left Carville or died, yet he changes rooms in Carville to have more space for his stuff. He inquires about the insurance money available to beneficiaries if something should happen to him, but in the same time frame offers to attend a conference in New Orleans to demonstrate his disease to others. Ultimately, Edmond spent the remainder of his days in Carville, but in February and March of 1928 this decision was not a certainty.

"We had a splendid trip to N.O." Edmond had volunteered to attend the conference in New Orleans to demonstrate his condition. In his February 28 letter to Dr. Denney, Edmond had even offered to generate leprosy symptoms including fever, pain, and tubercles.

It was at the New Orleans conference that Edmond met *"the man who was now in Carville expecting to be out in three weeks."* Remission and discharges from the hospital were rare in the 1920s and '30s, but new patients were often led to believe that they would be out in a matter of weeks. A series of tongue-in-cheek articles written by patients in the *Sixty Six Star* relate the adventures of Egbert, a naïve, fictional patient who entered the hospital expecting a quick and speedy recovery.

Carville, La.
June 11, 1928

Dear Folks:

I did not write last week because I had half way expected you all last Sunday and when you did not come Sunday I just put off writing.

I forgot to mention in my last letter about what you all ask about high water. The fact is that it is hard to know much about the roads in here. I have not heard anything about what you all inquired about. But last week [we] had a three days rain and believe me it did rain. We have a small lake on the back of the camp but after that rain the lake extended to the house next to mine, all the walks to the small cottages, owned by the patients in the back were under water. It is just about drained out now. It surely did stink for a few days when the water started to go down.

I also forgot to mention in my last letter that if Claire would not show you all my letter to let me know and I will mail you all a copy of it, for there is lots of things on it that I want you all to know, since she had brought you all also in our troubles.

I am now eating in the dining room again, and it does not seem to make any difference as I am still holding out about 200 #, and feeling well.

Hope that you all will be able to come before long.

Lots of love to all
As ever,
Edmond

Did you all mail the two letters I sent home the other day, I did not get any answer yet.

"*It is hard to know much about the roads . . .*" The roads into Carville were still unpaved at this time. Stanley Stein notes in the 1940s that it was a "miserable cart track that was an almost impassable river of mud in wet weather and a choking, bone-cracking nightmare of ruts and dust in the rest of the year" (230). Edmond by his own admission did not keep up with the news or weather of the area.

"*I also forgot to mention in my last letter that if Claire would not show you my entire letter . . .*" Two letters remain from the correspondence with Claire, one regarding the 1927 flood and a long, painful letter in June of 1928. Both of these letters are included in this chapter after his letters to his family to present what I see as the very different voice that Edmond uses when writing to his wife. The June 1928 letter is perhaps the one my grandfather references here, explaining why a copy of it remained. Claire either showed it to her in-laws who kept it or Edmond sent them a carbon copy of it.

[Thursday night: Undated] From this letter and the next dated August 27, 1928, it seems that Edmond must have visited New Iberia possibly to see Claire.

Dear Folks:—
We arrived here at 1 P.M. Had one puncture and missed one ferry connection.

Had dinner with Helen and Eddie and ate my chicken with them & the kids for supper. We all enjoyed them very much.

The trip did not tire me but Gee I am bluer, tonight, then I was before.

Lots of love to all
Edmond

....

Carville, La.
Aug 27, 1928

Dear Folks,
   I received Mamma's letter yesterday and was glad to hear from her.
   Glad that you all enjoyed my visit and I enjoyed it also even though things were not as I would have liked them but I expected such before leaving here. Don't you all say anything one way or the other. If Claire decides she wants to come here with you all I will let you all know. Hope she decides to. I've asked her to bring Mrs. Jones if she comes before you all do but she did not say anything about it. You don't have to worry about bringing her here for after she visits here she will leave her father's & go to her husband's people.
   We are expecting the California patients to-night. They reached NO after 8 P.M. to-night and will be here about 1 or 2 A.M. 5 Ladies and 7 men.
   I am not feeling too good to-night. I have a terrible headache. Guess I have been doing too much thinking lately.
   We are having a kind of storm to night so these patients coming from NO will have a pretty rough ride especially that they will have to drive slow on account of 2 of them are on stretchers.
   This is all for this time.

Lots of love to all.
As ever
Edmond

"Things were not as I would have liked . . ." Edmond had evidently re-turned to New Iberia for a visit, perhaps to achieve reconciliation with his

wife. They had not yet resolved their differences, but they were talking and Edmond was hopeful that Claire would visit him with the family.

"We are expecting the California patients . . ." Patients outside of Louisiana were often transported in locked train cars and served their meals on paper plates in their cars. Once in New Orleans they were transferred to ambulances to make the final trek on rough roads.

Oct 23, 1928

Dear Folks:—

I received Marie's letter (If I remember correctly it was Marie that wrote) and was glad to hear from her.

Our letters must have crossed last week as I did write and enclose a letter to be forwarded and I see that she received it.

I've been forgetting every time I write to ask you all to return me that long letter, so if you all are not coming before long please mail it to me.

I have not yet read the article from Brother E.

Love to all.
As ever
Edmond

"I've been forgetting . . ." It is possible that the long letter mentioned here is the June 1928 letter to my grandmother. I want to believe that my grandparents reconciled their differences and my grandfather did not want the letter further distributed. This is one of the last letters we have from my grandfather to his family until October 1929. Other letters could have been lost or destroyed, or relations with Claire had improved, and he wrote more letters to her which she may have shared with her in-laws but still did not keep (perhaps still fearing for the health of Booz and Teenie).

Saturday Morning [spring of 1929]

Dear Folks:——

I was to write last night but the school had a "commencement exercise" and my being in charge of the kids I had to be there. Was to get up early to write but did not sleep until 3 am so it was 6:45 when I woke up. So just a note whilst the mailman waits.

Sorry to hear that you all expect high water but I can't figure that way and if it does reach I can't figure that it will be very high. You all can write and tell me after it is all over. All this is God's will and I can't help at all so the less I know about it when it is going on the less worry it will be to me and for that reason I don't read any papers nor listen on the radio.

I have asked the Sisters to pray for you all and they said they would.

I was elected president of the Club this week and am feeling alright.

Lots of love to all
As ever
Edmond

"*Commencement exercises . . .*" According to Julia Elwood, a former patient at Carville, teacher in the hospital school, and editor of the centennial booklet *Known Simply to the Rest of the World as Carville*, "The School was started in 1940. . . . It was an accredited school" (56). I can't explain the discrepancy since my grandfather's letter seems to indicate some type of educational ceremony. Perhaps the earlier school in the 1920s was for youth only and non-accredited. The later school was for adults as well as youth and was accredited. Education had been a value at Carville since the earliest days when the Daughters of Charity would teach and read to the patients.

"*I was elected president of the Club . . .*" apparently refers to the "What Cheer Club."

Carville, La. Oct 13, 1929

Dear Folks,

 I received Marie's letter to-day and was very glad to hear from her and especially to know that mamma was alright again. Hope this will be her last attack.

 Tell her to try those tablets for her pains in her arm also. She does not have to wait for a bad headache.

 How did the pictures you all took here come out? Get me two of each and mail them to me letting me know how much.

 Also mail to

Mrs. W. D. Skipper

Marion, S.C.

5# Large Pecans and to

Mrs. C. Stappenbeck

2721 S. Prieur St.

New Orleans, La.

10# Lge Pecans

Send both by insured mail and let me know how much

Sr R[egina] was glad to learn that mama is alright again and sends her best regards to all.

 I am not in charge of the boys any longer. They have been put in men's houses, all of them. I still hold the oil job, and like it better that way.

 My cold is all gone and I feel alright.

Lots of love to all.

As ever

Edmond

[PS]How is Tante Eugenie with her smothering spell?

"*Also mail to . . .*" Pecans were plentiful on the Landry property in New Iberia and Edmond requested them for patients and their families during more than one season. There were also pecan trees in Carville, but perhaps the patients themselves were hesitant to send pecans from the hospital grounds to their families, or the families were afraid to eat them, or shipping packages from the hospital was difficult.

"*I am not in charge of the boys* . . ." Edmond had been in charge of the young boys at Carville from 1925–1929. His rules for them (page 129) indicate that he was a strict disciplinarian. In 1929, he was released from his duties for reasons that are not totally clear. See page 135 for his discussion of this in a letter to Dr. Denney.

"*I still hold the oil job* . . ." Edmond evidently distributed the chaulmoogra oil capsules to patients. Stanley Stein, who held the same job in the 1930s, notes that patients could request the number of pills that they wanted. One patient often asked for a seemingly unusual number of them. When Stein inquired about the use of the pills, the patient explained that he used the extra capsules to grease his hair. Other patients admitted that the extra pills were sent home to relatives who had the disease but feared going to the hospital (56–57).

Carville, La
Nov. 29, 1929

Dear Folks,
   I received Marie's letter and was glad to hear from her.
   I also received the Buttons and they will do alright. Keep account and will pay on your next visit.
   Glad that you all are getting good results on your radio. We have a set in our house. We boys bought it $125.00 only but the best I heard yet. Tune in on W.L.W. 6:15 PM "Tony's Scrap Book." I like it as it is always a good phylosophy. We get about 80 different stations on our set.
   Last Nov. you remember I burnt my left hand. This Nov. I burnt my right. But not much. Looks as if it is only during this month that I burn. I am O.K. and have not had but one headache in more than two months. Still weigh 197#.
   We had a very nice Thanksgiving Day yesterday and as bad as some things are we have lots to be thankful for.

Lots of love and best wishes to all.
As ever
Edmond

"Glad that you all are getting good results on your radio. We have a set . . ."
According to my mother, the family radio was one that Edmond had given
them. She remembers her uncle and his friends crowding around it to listen
to the boxing matches. The radio that the "boys" bought may have been
set up in a common area that was part of each house. Patients had private
rooms in a house holding about 12 patients and a common area that allowed
for visiting and recreation. This was the beginning of the Great Depression
and $125.00 would have been a considerable outlay of money for men with
few sources of income.

"Last Nov. you remember . . ." Burns were a hazard for HD patients who
often lost feeling in their extremities and were thus subject to accidents with
cigarettes, hot water, or cooking appliances. Edmond's brother, Albert, recalled holding a cigarette that was burning his fingers, but he did not know
he was being injured until someone pointed it out to him. In some cases,
unheeded damages to extremities could become infected leading to further
problems and sometimes amputations.

3/30/30

Dear Folks:—
    *Received Amelie's letter and was glad to know that mamma was
resting nicely and doing well. Hope it will continue. Tell her I'll
make my Easter Duties.*
    *Sr. R. was sorry to hear about her being sick, also the other Sisters
and they all send mamma their best wishes and told me to tell her
they are praying for her.*
    I am enclosing a few dollars to help out with the bill.
    I am doing well and very busy as it is the end of the month.
    *Mailing letters in afternoon is too late as it delays them 24 hours.
Tell mamma I'll write her when she is resting easier.*

Lots of love to all.
Edmond

"Tell her I'll make my Easter Duties." This is the first acknowledgment
that Edmond had returned to the sacraments of the Catholic Church.
Evidently whatever impediment had prevented him from receiving
Communion had been resolved and Edmond had received absolution.

4/4/30

Dear Folks: —

I have received the letters but they don't come regularly every day. One day I get two, next day none that is because you all don't mail them before the 1ˢᵗ train which goes by home about 11:00 am. A letter on the 2 pm train doesn't always get here the next day.

Glad to hear that mama is doing so well and hope she will be herself again soon. Hope the gas trouble and her vein trouble have left her.

I sent a registered letter from here Monday. Did you all get it? I address so many of my letters to N.O. instead of N.I. that since you all did not mention having received same it may have gone to N.O. I forgot to inquire about Amelie's burned face and she has not said any more about it. Hope it is well by now.

I am going to have a Mass said next week in thanks for mama's speedy recovery and will take communion for Easter Duties as stated in my previous letter.

Glad that Claire went to see mama.

I want you all to see Edmond and ask him, if he would allow me to see mama at the hospital for one visit someday next week, as a patient from here went up that way this week and they are going back to get him next week so I could stop on the way up. Tell him not to hesitate to say "No" if he is the least bit skeptical, for if he allows me to visit I don't want any red tape or string but to be allowed to enter his hospital like any other person.

Give my love to mamma and tell her I am praying for her.

Lots of love to all.
As ever,
Edmond

"*I sent a registered letter . . .*" In the collection of letters and artifacts from Carville there is a registered envelope postmarked March 31, 1930, and addressed to Miss Amelie Landry. Markings on it indicate that it was sent incorrectly to New Orleans. The return address on the letter was "Gabe Michael, Carville, La." My mother always contended that neither her mother nor her father used the name Gabe Michael in correspondence.

Perhaps it is used here since it was a registered letter from Carville and may have contained the money mentioned in the March 30 letter.

"I forgot to inquire about Amelie's burned face . . ." Amelie manifested symptoms of leprosy as early as 1923 even though she did not enter the hospital until 1934. Loss of feeling (especially in hands and feet) is one of the effects of the condition. I do not know if her burned face would also have been because of leprosy.

"I want you all to see Edmond . . ." Dr. Edmond Landry was Lucie Landry's godson and a New Iberia doctor who tended to her. My grandfather asserts his agency requesting permission to visit his mother in the New Iberia hospital, like anyone else.

"A patient from here went up that way . . ." Travel restrictions for Carville patients were relaxing, especially for those in Louisiana and Texas, but patients still needed permission from the Board of Health of each state through which they traveled.

[This undated letter, simply marked "Wednesday A.M.," indicates that Edmond did get permission to visit his mother in the hospital.]

Wednesday A.M.

Dear Folks:—

We arrived here safe and sound last night at 7:10. Just in time for the show.

Don't feel very tired this morning.

Sorry I did not get to see Edmond yesterday but thank him for me.

Hope Mamma is still feeling alright and that she is getting rid of her gas. Sr. R. says maybe she does not eat enough solid food.

Must get this off.

Lots of love to all
As ever
Edmond

July 16, 1930

Dear Folks:—

   Just a note this morning to let you all know that poor John W. died last night. Sr. R. was with him and he just died in his sleep. She was supposed to send for me but she could not locate watchman and when the end came he went fast. Poor fellow he is far better off.

   I am feeling fine and hope all's well at home.

As ever
Edmond

....

[Sept. 14, 1931]
Saturday Morning

Dear Folks:—

   I received Marie's letter and was very glad to hear from you all and to know you all had made the trip back home OK.

   Was sorry but not surprised to hear about aunt Mimmie's death. Hope uncle Eraste won't take it too hard. As long as she could not recover, she is better off now than to continue her suffering. Extend to Uncle Eraste and the family my sincere sympathy and condolence

   We enjoyed the chicken and cake very much but the chicken, as good as it tasted sure did make us sick. Val, Alice, and I should not have opened it at the house and not take it out the can. Will know better next time. I first thought it was my cramps of the week before getting worse but when I found out Val & Alice were sick too, then I knew it was the chicken. Sr. R. fussed at me the next day for not having gone to hospital. I told her I wanted to go but could not. I was sitting on back porch—House 41—talking to Felix feeling alright and all of a sudden my stomach felt funny and I just made it to the sink. That was 9:30 P.M. and I never left until midnight and when I felt better it was no use going to hospital. Am feeling O.K. Hope all of you are well.

Lots of love to all.
Edmond

"Val, Alice and I should not have opened it . . ." It is not clear where Val, Alice, and Edmond ate the chicken. Perhaps they ate in Edmond's cottage or in one of the houses. Men and women lived in separate houses and the men were prohibited from going into the women's rooms. Patients managed to circumvent the rule by setting up a card table in the doorway of a room, with the man sitting in the hall to play cards or to enjoy meals together.

[3-19-32]
Saturday Morn

Dear Folks,
 I received Mamma's letter and was glad to hear from her.
 We had a 16 reel show last night and it lasted too late so I did not write last night.
 It is perfectly alright with me about what mamma asked, I can get another from U.S.
 I am feeling alright and waiting for the trees.
 Hope all of you are well

Lots of love to all
Edmond

....

Monday Night
4—12—32

Dear Folks:—
 I received Marie's letter yesterday. Glad to hear from her. Sorry she is sick but hope will be alright when this letter reaches you all.
 About the mysterious letter, I knew there was no chance for her to enter here on such "mission" but I spoke to Sister Martha about it anyway. She says for mamma to tell her she can not get work here but if she really wants work she should take it up with some Foreign Mission Society that does lots of good work in foreign colonies, but she can take it from me it's a hard life.

Sr. Katherine told me once that she frequently gets such requests. I think it might be someone who has this and is trying to get here on a blind to the public.

I am doing a little better. I don't cough as much and my throat is not as sore.

Hope you all are well.

Lots of love to all.
As ever
Edmond

"*About the mysterious letter . . .*" In the family collection there is an anonymous letter to Mrs. Landry, Edmond's mother, asking for information about entering the religious life, specifically the Daughters of Charity. The writer goes to great lengths to insure anonymity, requesting that any information be sent to a post office box identified only by a box number. My grandfather's assessment of the letter is plausible and if it is correct it reiterates the fear of stigmatization faced by those suffering with leprosy.

Saturday AM
[August 27, 1932]

Dear Folks:——

Was glad to hear you all had gotten back home without much trouble. Don't think it rained here the day you all were here but we have had some nearly every day since. It is good for each rain brings us cool weather.

The "66 Star" (Local Paper) today [August 27, 1932] had an answer to the one on the States about this place. It is a hot one and I'll give it to Claire when she comes next week and you all can get it when she is through reading it. And there is a very good article by Dr. McCoy.

3 Patients are to be discharged this week—Sidney H. is one of them.

I am feeling fine these days and hope all of you are well.

Lots of love to all
As ever
Edmond

"The '66 Star' today had an answer . . ." James P. Walsh, Special Correspondent for the *New Orleans States*, had written an article about the "idyllic" conditions of Carville: lush surroundings, patients happy to return to the institution, and paid employment for patients able to work. David H. Palmer, a patient, issued a signed and stinging rebuttal to the article in the *Sixty Six Star*. Palmer disputed the veracity of Walsh's article, noting rather sardonically that allegedly a picture of George Washington had fallen from the wall and tears were detected in his eyes when the article was read aloud in the Carville library. Palmer's greatest objection to the article was the Pollyanna view it portrayed and its failure to recognize that for those living unwillingly within the confines of the hospital, Carville was not a paradise, but a cage.

"Sidney H. is one of them." By this time the Landry family had been visiting Carville for more than ten years and must have been familiar with many of the patients there.

[The remaining letters to his "Folks" were undated; the bracketed dates were determined from internal evidence or from tentative dates on the envelopes in which they were originally found.]

[November 12, 1931]

Dear Folks:—

I did not write to Claire yesterday as it was a holiday and no mail went out.

Was glad to hear that Albert was better and hope he is O.K. by now and that no one else will get this flu.

I am feeling fairly well but there is always something that aches. This morning it is a new gland under my left arm

Will you all have enough pecans to mail out for me as ordered last year. If so let me know and I'll send the list.

A new patient came in yesterday. A boy 10—Brother to one of the girls here. I did not see him but they tell me the poor kid is in very bad shape already.

The play by the patients last night was perfect and everybody enjoyed it.

Hope all of you are well

Love to all
Edmond

"*There is always something that aches.*" Although my grandfather had not complained much during his early years at Carville, by 1931 he was in and out of the hospital and mentioned more aches, pains, and swollen glands.

"*A new patient came in yesterday . . . very bad shape . . .*" Leprosy has never been considered hereditary and it is only mildly contagious, but there were at Carville families who had more than one member with the disease. That Edmond mentions the boy's very bad condition again points out that patients often tried to avoid entrance to Carville for as long as possible.

"*The play by the patients . . .*" Stanley Stein entered Carville in the spring of 1931 and by November had organized a Little Theater presentation by the patients. This was the first such theatrical event. Sister Laura had directed musical pageants for several years and Edmond had organized a minstrel earlier in 1931.

Sat. A.M.
[10–22–32]

Dear Folks:——

I received Marie's letter with my check and was glad to hear from her.

Everything here is on a dead stop. The only news we have lately is that they have measured off the grounds for the new hospital again but it looks as if they mean business this time. It is not going to be wards but will be 65 rooms. That will help as the rooms are nearly all taken up.

I have been enjoying the nice weather lately and feel better from it.

Hope all of you are well

Lots of love to all
As ever
Edmond

"Everything here is on a dead stop . . . measured off the ground for the new hospital . . ." It had been sixteen months since the Carville veterans had met with Sam Jones to get more support and recognition for the institution. The country was in the midst of the depression and movement was slow but eventually some progress was being made. The hospital was coming along, although Edmond did not live to see its completion. By 1934, when Amelie entered Carville, the hospital had been completed and more activity had begun.

Sat. AM
[11–5–32]

Dear Folks,

Just a note. I had a bad gas attack that kept me awake nearly all night. Got 2 hours sleep and just woke up feeling OK but sore & tired.

Must hurry to catch mail man Love to all

Edmond

"*I had a bad gas attack that kept me awake . . .*" This is three weeks before my grandfather entered the infirmary for the last time and one month before his death.

Sat. A.M.
[11–25–32; Edmond entered the infirmary on 11–27–32 for the last time.]

Dear Folks:—
   Just a few lines to say that I am better this morning. I was suffering too much to write to Claire yesterday. It was just a gland under my left arm that got almost as big as my head and believe me it hurt. I did not sleep a wink Thursday night but did get some sleep last night. The gland is gone down considerably and it does not pain me much so I guess I'll be alright. It can't be much for with all that, I did not have fever but it has killed my appetite and left me weak. I could not eat a thing on Thanksgiving Day, as good a dinner as we had only drank milk and that would come up.
   Hope all of you are O.K.

Lots of love to all
As ever
Edmond

[The following letters to Edmond's family are undated and lack any clear evidence to suggest accurate dates for them. However, most of them do seem to reflect my grandfather's failing health, so they may have been written during the last months of his life.]

Friday Night

Dear Folks:—

   Just a few lines to let you all have of my news which are good. The glands in my neck have all gone and I feel fine and I am enjoying the cool breeze that came up this morning.

   I have been getting letters from Claire regularly and they are making the trip O.K and they expect to be back home somewhere around next Sunday.

   Everything here is about the same.

   Hope all of you are well.

Lots of love to all
As ever
Edmond

....

Friday Night

Dear Folks:

   Received Marie's letter to-day and was glad to hear from her and to know all of you are well.

   I am expecting Claire to-morrow.

   Please Ship 5# pecans to each of the following addresses

Mrs. W. D. Skipper 44 cents
Marion, S.C.

Mrs. C. Stappenbeck
630 Toledano St. 17 cents
New Orleans, La.

5 # to me

Mr. Wm H. Collins 83 cents
#3 Fletcher Lane
Key West, Fla.

Miss Josie Cuccia
3500 Dryades St. 17 cents
New Orleans, La.

Send the large ones and keep track of all charges and I'll pay
when you all come next time.
I am feeling a little better and my last kidney test showed much
improvement again.
Hope all of you are well.

Lots of love to all
As ever
Edmond

....

Tuesday Night

Dear Folks,
Just a few words to say I am about the same. Still in bed. Wanted
to get up to-day but it was too cold. My feet and legs are still swollen.
Hope all the sick are alright by now.
Will play Santa Claus when you all come.
Merry Xmas to you all at Lafayette and at uncle H.

Love to all
Edmond

....

Friday Night

Dear Folks:—
Well I am still in bed and in my room feeling a little better. Ate a
little more to-day. My sore tongue is still doing better. My strength
is slow coming back.
Hope mama's cold and fever is all gone by now.
Phone Claire give her of my news.

Lots of love to all
As ever
Edmond

Carville, La.
Apr. 28, 1927.

Dear Claire:—
Well the river situation is not getting any better. They claim we are safe but I found out to-night there is seapage not far from the big gate and from the little I know about levee's—seapage is not very good. If the things gets worse and breaks well you all — you and the folks — come to get me and my gang. I'll pay all expenses. You know I never liked

In April 1927, Edmond acknowledged his fear for himself and the other patients in Carville if the levee were to break. (Landry Letters from Carville; used with permission.)

Letters from Carville—Dear Claire

"Let me know by return mail what I must expect if the worse comes."
Edmond to Claire, April 1927

The next two letters, one from April 28, 1927, and another, undated but apparently from early June 1928, are the only two letters remaining in my grandfather's correspondence with my grandmother, but they are far more disturbing than the entire collection to his family. The anger and pain that he only rarely and obliquely mentioned to his family are poured out to his wife. With her he could request the support he needed, and write of the fears he had and the abiding love he felt for her. He also acknowledged the anguish and disappointment that was his because of her physical and emotional distance from him. The closing on those two letters is more abrupt, but here too he is "as ever" husband and father, a man passionately in love with the woman he prayed for all his life and longing for the love she seems unable to return.

We have always assumed that the letters from my grandfather were destroyed by my grandmother because of her fear of leprosy and her desire to protect herself and her children from the ravages of the disease. My mother recalls that her mother would read the letters, carefully edited, to her and her brother, but that they never touched nor read them for themselves. The contents of the longest remaining letter from my grandfather to my grandmother reveal the discord that existed between my grandparents for a time and suggests that my grandmother may have destroyed the letters from her husband to protect the children from the turmoil she and my grandfather were living. The first of the two surviving letters mentions Edmond's parents specifically so it may have been shared with them. The second, more damning letter may have been sent by Edmond himself to his parents since they had become cognizant of the problems between my grandparents. This would explain its survival.

Carville, La.
Apr. 28, 1927

Dear Claire:—

Well the river situation is not getting any better. They claim we are safe but I found out to-night there is seepage not far from the big gate and from the little I know about levees—seepage is not very good. If the thing gets worse and breaks will you all—you and the folks—come to get me and my gang. I'll pay all expenses.

You know I never liked levees anyway and now being a "leper" I wonder just how much rescue help would come to us in distress and as close as I can figure it the majority will say let them drown, its good riddance. Like Sr. M[artha] told me when they operated on the baby. They were to chloroform him so I told her to have his heart examined before as his pulse was 175 to 200 and she replied— Gabe don't worry it would be a blessing if he died. Well it may be a blessing to us to be taken out of our misery but I be dam if I want to be murdered. All those things make me so mad that I don't know myself.

Many thanks for the Easter Egg.

Don't get excited and phone authorities here they will tell you like they tell us "Everything is OK" but they got a boat in front the big house, for their use.
Let me know by return mail what I must expect if the worse comes.

Edmond

"Well the river situation is not getting any better . . ." The flood of 1927 was one that is still recognized today for the social, political, geographic, and cultural upheaval it wrought. The United States Public Health Hospital at Carville was ultimately not affected, but this letter suggests the fear that the patients experienced. Edmond's account of the threat of flooding in Carville presents more than a breach in the levee; it indicates the unreachable divide between personnel and patients. The patients were well taken care of by the federal, religious, and lay personnel, and the narrative that endures even today is that the hospital was ready to evacuate,

but the perception of the patients seemed to be different. There was still more than a hedge between patients and the staff. In a 1984 interview with Marcia Gaudet, Sister Laura Stricker, who had been at Carville in 1927, gives credence to Edmond's distress. "In 1927, we had the high water, and we had to use sandbags to hold the water. They had a barge out there, and they had men on the barge all night long. And if the levee would break, they were supposed to bring the patients out of the hospital and on to the barge. There were handicapped people who couldn't walk/and some were blind; and if they would have had to get them out of there— I don't think they would have made it" (*Remembering Carville*, 181–82). Personally I wonder what would have happened had a rescue from the hospital been successful. Would the refugee centers have accepted leprosy patients into their midst?

"Come to get me and my gang." Edmond was in charge of the young boys until 1929. He clearly felt a deep responsibility and affection for them.

"The majority will say let them drown, its good riddance." I cannot prove that there was a factual basis to my grandfather's statement, but it clearly shows the emotion of a man who felt his life and that of other leprosy patients was expendable. My grandfather is disturbed at the attitude toward his life, the lives of the other patients, and that of this obviously sick baby. Although the situations were separate, they both affected my grandfather profoundly. It might be a blessing if they died, but he does not want to be murdered. The sick baby in question may have been a newborn in need of some kind of surgery. In my grandfather's view, he, too, was due a chance at life. Babies born to female patients in Carville were routinely taken from their mothers and put in foster homes or in the orphanage in New Orleans run by the Daughters of Charity. The presence of my grandfather in the baby's treatment corroborates other evidence that patients helped with deliveries.

"Don't get excited and phone authorities here . . ." I never knew my grandfather, but these words capture my grandmother well and indicate the relation between them, illustrated by the familiarity my grandfather had with my grandmother's reaction.

A FINAL SURVIVING LETTER

> *"For nearly four long years I have begged you to treat me better than you have."*
> Edmond to his wife, ca. June 1928

This next letter deserves some context for its very existence. In 1928, Edmond may have sent a copy of it to his parents after he had sent it to Claire. He seems to have asked for its return but that was not done and the letter remained in my great-grandmother Lucie's collection of letters. In 1977, it was saved by Paul, Booz, and Teenie, along with all the other letters and mementos in Albert's small apartment. When Martin Landry, Paul's brother and Edmond's second grandson, began organizing the letters, he decided to separate this one and one other letter, still lost, from the collection. As he explained at the time, he separated these from the larger collection in deference to our grandmother who was still alive, because of our love for her, and because the letters were "tough to read." In 1977, I knew about the letter but at the time chose not to read it. My own life was in transition: my relationship with my grandmother was central to me, and I was not ready to have my image of her challenged. I knew that both Martin and my brother Michael had copies of the long mysterious letter and I remained naively confident that it would be there if and when I ever wanted to read it.

My life continued, but always in the back of my mind I knew that the collection of letters (including this one) would be available to me when I wanted to read it. When I finally read the collection of my grandfather's letters in 1998, I inquired about the "long letter," for I felt it would fill in some gaps in my grandfather's correspondence and explain comments that he made to his parents and siblings. Michael and Martin had only vague recollections of it and neither one had success in finding the letter. Twenty-two years had passed since it was first discovered. The busyness, joys, and heartaches of life had moved the letter from their consciousness and the accumulations of life had pushed it deep into storage.

Despite its loss, I continued with my studies, convinced that the letter had indeed been irrevocably lost or destroyed. In my work, I discovered the grandfather I had searched for as a child. I completed my work and graduated in December 2007, comfortable that I had an accurate image of my grandfather. On a Sunday morning in March 2008, almost three months to the day after my graduation, my brother called, "Claire, we found the letter." When

I received my copy of it, I excitedly anticipated reading it, but I was stopped cold by my grandfather's first line, "For nearly four long years I have begged you to treat me better than you have."

The letter was tougher than anything I had imagined. It surpassed the anguish I had envisaged for my grandfather, and it put to the test the experience I had of my grandmother: frightened of leprosy, but constant in her love of her husband. My mother had on occasion mentioned that her parents had "had some difficulty," but this letter told of more than that. The letter was full of raw pain and accusations from my grandfather, lonely and isolated from his wife and children. It poured out his anger and pain, but it also expressed the profound injustice he felt, incarcerated for a misunderstood and unfairly feared condition. His grief throbbed through the close, tightly typed, single-spaced, eighteen-page letter, making it impossible for me to read in a single sitting. I skimmed it at first, trying to prepare myself for its onslaught. Finally, I decided to retype the letter, double-spaced for easier reading. The slow, tedious recopying became for me an introductory meditation into the turmoil in my grandparents' lives, and the typing initially shielded me from the full impact of the letter's stark reality. It gave me new insight into my grandfather's life in Carville and forced me to see him as desperately human and stripped of any façade. It also made me admit that human love is not always perfect love and it obliged me to accept that for a number of years my grandmother could not or did not find the kind of love for her husband that he so desperately needed. I, no longer a child, was forced to accept not just mythical, idealized grandparents separated by fear and disease, but a man and a woman struggling across an abyss. My grandfather, lonely and cognizant of the injustice of his incarceration, begged for his wife's love. My grandmother, fearful of leprosy, its stigma, and the risk to their children, was paralyzed, unable to meet her husband's powerful request.

The act of embracing this particular letter has been difficult for my brothers and cousins, as well as for me. We knew our grandmother; she was flesh, blood, and unconditional love for us from infancy into adulthood. Her home and heart were always open; her pantry was always stocked with our favorite treats, with cold Coca-Cola always in the refrigerator, and often a "little change" on the dresser for each of us. She was the constant in our lives. Hers was the home of refuge and escape from the usual issues between parents and siblings. Although she was not a demonstrative woman, she was a loving, steadfast grandmother, and at her funeral each of her seven grandsons was surprised to discover that he was not her favorite. As the only girl, I am still convinced that I was her favorite, but the evidence is that she loved each of us truly, unconditionally, and uniquely, and we still take comfort in that.

Understandably, this deep love we felt for "Mamman" made accepting our grandfather's letter difficult for us. We seem incapable even today of talking about it without using euphemisms. It is still referred to as "the eighteen-page letter" or just "The Letter." We have chosen to accept the letter in different ways: a refusal to read it, a conviction that that is "not Mamman," a sense that her fear of leprosy had controlled her and that this explains her actions. I have taken consolation in the fact that my grandparents were reconciled; my grandfather did not leave Carville, as he threatened, and there is evidence after 1928 that my grandmother did again visit my grandfather. She was also present at his bedside on the day he died, having been called there at his request. We will never know the full outcome of this letter that arrests time with such painful memories. Perhaps my grandmother subsumed her fear and visited my grandfather as his wife, or my grandfather reconciled himself to the companionship that his wife was willing to give, but I do know that the letter as it stands speaks loudly of the pain of my grandfather and so many others whose lives were overshadowed by leprosy.

More than eighty years after it was written, this letter still holds passion and power. If it is difficult for me to read even now, I can only imagine the pain it caused my grandparents. Earlier letters to my great-grandparents indicate that there had been discord between my grandfather and grandmother before 1928, so the letter was not a complete surprise to my grandmother. According to my mother, at some point, my grandmother's hair turned completely grey overnight; this letter could have done that. It was an ultimatum she may have dreaded but never expected. Edmond presented his carefully researched facts about leprosy; his conviction that his disease was not a threat to her; that her visits to Carville would not threaten their children; and his utter loneliness without his family. The decision was now Claire's to make. Would fear or love rule her life?

My grandmother's fear was overwhelming and understandable. Her husband was the second in his family to be incarcerated in Carville. Her youngest sister-in-law, Amelie, had already shown signs of leprosy. Claire had two young children, ages nine and six, who she feared were susceptible to leprosy. Her own mother had a morbid fear of dirt, germs, bacteria, and contagion of any kind. The disease was incurable and could cause horrific disfigurement and scarring. Intellectually, my grandmother had known about leprosy since Norbert entered Carville; she baked cookies and sent novenas to him, but she confronted the reality of the disease when it entered her home in 1922, the time of Edmond's first diagnosis. Between 1922 and 1924, she must have made some emotional truce with this intruder that had sickened her husband and threatened their children. She confronted the full ravages of leprosy for the first time when she visited her husband at the hospital. Only then did she personally witness the wreckage the disease could cause to some patients: gnarled and numb limbs, blinded eyes, the identity changing horrors to faces, the stench and grim forbearance of patients imprisoned like criminals and doomed to die. Revulsion would have been a natural human instinct. Carville was not a place she wanted to enter and the condition was not one she wished on their children. As much as she loved her husband, she would have done anything in her power to save Teenie and Booz from this fate and to protect them from seeing their father perhaps disfigured before their eyes. Up until June of 1928, nothing had penetrated her fear. From medical science we now know that her fear was irrational, but in 1928 for her it was real.

Edmond, however, had of necessity faced his fear. He was the unspeakable, he was a "leper," but he was also a man who desperately wanted the woman he loved, and he made his arguments to his wife. I imagine he struggled with numb fingers and deep depression to marshal the most current scientific research, medical evidence, anecdotal accounts, and his own frustration into a plea to his wife. He may first have handwritten the letter, editing and amending it before he finally laboriously typed multiple carbon copies of the eighteen-page missive giving his wife a last chance to accept him, leaving it to Claire to decide their fate.

I don't have my grandmother's answer or further letters between my grandparents, but love did prevail, as somehow my grandfather and grandmother made accommodations that eventually enabled them to have a relationship until his death

I have transcribed the content of the letter in its entirety, making a few bracketed notes for clarity, and adding bracketed subtitles as transition. The initials "EGL," for Edmond Gilbert Landry, were my grandfather's own insertions and indicate specific comments initialed by him. Otherwise the letter stands as written.

Dear Claire :
                          nearly
          For four long years I have begged you to treat me better than
you have and for the last two years of these four I have tried to, in a
way, force you to come, thinking that you had enough love for me that
such long absence would have made you long for me as it has made me long
for you but all has been in vain. For two long years I've put off writing
this letter to you always hoping that you would have come to your senses
and seen this disease in the same light that I do, especially, after all
that I told you about it that no one else knows but you think that I am
crazy and view these fact from that stand point because I am a leper and
you still want to be parted from me as you have for the past six years,
this month, in spite of the fact that you now know that I was a leper
before we married(and I since have Dr. Denny's statement at N. O. that I
have leprosy 15 years with a probable incubation period of 7 years) but
I now know that I have it 32 years and will someday prove it) and as I've
told you before your actions have made me want to disappear but before
doing this I want to recall lots of facts that I have already told you &
tell you many more that I had never mentioned and also give you statements

from prominent Doctors to corroborate mine and if you still refuse to
visit me as my wife, at least, once a month I will then enter where I have
tried hard to keep from but where I will then know that I belong in the
"land of the unmarried dead"
          Before I start with making statements, etc., I want you to know
that all this is hurting me more than it is you for I am forced to follow
the road that I am in whilst your path which you claim is not all roses
is followed at your own wishes. You were the best wife that a man ever
could wish for and I've loved the very grounds that you walked on. I had,
eversince a young boy, prayed   daily for a good
wife and after finding you I thought that my prayers were answered and
thanked God every day until I was here for some time when I found out
that you would not have me for "better or worse" but that you were with
rest of the prejudiced public and majority of wives who think that the
unwritten law of marriage is "Until death or leprosy do us part", and
many are the nights that I have spent sleepless thinking about the injustice of your still wanting to be parted from me and refusing me one
day per month after you having lived as close to me as you did for the
years that you did,when I was more of a leper than I am now and which
fact I will to prove to you and if you still refuse to come back to me
than I will be free and blameless for my future actions.
          Claire, you know that when I found out I had leprosy and was pro-
mised by Dr. Roussell to be cured in two years, we agreed to live as
brother and sister; not that I thought it was a real necessity but just
to please you for any one who loved you as I did would have made that
"sacrifice" for the loving wife that I thought you were. How to prove
the unnecessariness of this I will recall to you Dr. Roussell's statement to me when he said I had leprosy; "You have had this for
nine years and if you have not infected any one during that time why
should ye infect anyone now! (Now you add 6 years to these 9 years and you
will see where Dr. D. is not so far wrong) We also have Dr. Sabatier's

First page of an eighteen-page letter. Eighty years have not dimmed the anguish of this tightly typed 1928 letter by Edmond pleading with Claire to show her love and visit him as his wife. (Landry Letters from Carville; used with permission.)

Dear Claire:

[COME TO ME AS I HAVE BEGGED YOU] *For nearly four long years I have begged you to treat me better than you have and for the last two of these four I have tried to, in a way, force you to come, thinking that you had enough love for me that such long absence would have made you long for me as it has made me long for you but all has been in vain. For two long years I've put off writing this letter to you always hoping that you would have come to your senses and seen this discussion in the same light that I do, especially after all that I told you about it that no one else knows, but you think that I am crazy and view these facts from that stand point because I am a "leper" and you still want to be parted from me as you have for the past six years, this month in spite of the fact that you now know that I was a "leper" before we got married (and I since have Dr. Denny's statement at N.O. that I have leprosy 15 years with a probable incubation period of 7 years, but I now know that I have it 32 [years] and will someday prove it) and as I've told you before your actions have made me want to disappear but before doing this I want to recall lots of facts that I have already told you and tell you many more that I had never mentioned and also give you statements from prominent Doctors to corroborate mine and if you still refuse to visit me as my wife, at least, once a month I will then enter where I tried hard to keep from but where I will then know that I belong in the "land of the unburied dead."*

Before I start with making statements, etc., I want you to know that all this is hurting me more than it is you for I am forced to follow the road that I am on whilst your path which you claim "is not all roses" is followed at your own wishes. You were the best wife that a man ever could wish for and I've loved the very grounds that you walked on. I had, ever since a young boy, prayed daily for a good wife and after finding you I thought that my prayers were answered and thanked God every day until I was here for some time when I found out that you would not have me for "better or worse" But that you were with the rest of the prejudiced public and majority of wives who think that the unwritten law of marriage is "until death or leprosy do us part" [spouses of leprosy patients had a legal right to file for divorce] *and many are the nights that I have spent sleepless thinking about the injustice of your still wanting to be parted from me and refusing me one day per month after you have lived so close to me as you did for the years that you did, when I was more of a "leper" than I am now and which fact I will prove to you and if you still refuse to come back to me then I will be free and blameless for my future actions.*

Claire, you know that when I found out I had leprosy [1922] and was promised by Dr. Roussell to be cured in two years, we agreed to live as brother and sister; not that I thought it was a real necessity but just to please you for anyone who loved you as I did would have made that "sacrifice" for the loving wife that I thought you were. Now to prove the unnecessariness of this I will recall to you Dr. Roussell's statement to me when he said I had leprosy; "You have had this for nine years and you have not infected anyone during that time [why] should you infect anyone now" (Now you add 6 years to those 9 years and you will see where Dr. D. is not so far wrong). We also have Dr. Sabatier's statement that "A 'leper' with an open sore could rub that sore against the sore of a healthy person and that person would not be infected unless he was susceptible to the disease." He proved that he was not scared of the disease when I had all those open tubercules and he would sit in my room on my bed and scratch his arm with prickly heat on it. Dr. Mayo from Mayo Bros. [Clinic] told two men here that they could go any where they wanted that they could not infect any one but that they [the doctors] had to report their case to their State Board of Health but that they would not do so immediately and they did not notify them [the Board of Health] until two months later, giving them [the two men] all the time they wanted to change towns or state. [Federal law required that leprosy cases be reported to public health. Doctors though used their discretion on this point.] *I have not any open sore and have not had any in three years. I am in far better health to-day than I was all the days I lived with you. New Iberia Board of Health I guess is patting itself on the back for having all infectious disease under control including the only case of leprosy in the parish, therefore thinking that there is no more danger from that source but I can go home and pick out 10 "lepers" off the streets in worse shape than I am and one of them has done work for you since I am here. My going home, I could not give it to any one for every one knows that I have it but these they don't know it themselves. I don't want to go home by absconding as I had first intended but I do want to be visited and treated as a living man instead of a corpse at a wake, as all of your several visits here were, which were more heart rendering [than] cheerful. If the disease would come on suddenly and you did not know that I had it before we married I would not ask you to visit me in this way, but I do insist that one or two days visits per month would not infect you now, if the long years of close contact of married life, as close as we were to each other did not already infect you. If you have been infected during those long years since you now fear the danger of one day, what difference does it make if you do expose yourself to it now. Whether you visit me or not, will not prevent you from developing it in years from now if you have to have it. Just as I have told Sr. M.[Martha] if I knew that my being here would prevent you and the kids from having leprosy, I would be contented to stay but I feel sure that one of you will have it in the future so what is the good of isolation.* [Neither Edmond's wife, children, grandchildren, great-grandchildren, or great-great-grandchildren have ever contracted HD.] *She said, well why do you stay here since you feel this way. Because if I went home and later on my kid or kids developed leprosy which is for them to have, whether I am home or not, the kids and the public would accuse me of being a low down no count for having infected them. A lady here, developed leprosy some years ago when her baby was two years old and the board of health at once sent her here to protect her baby, who was two years old. Eleven years later this baby, a boy now 13 years old, was recognized to be a "leper" and was sent here. He is the picture of health but last year he had a sore on his hand and the parents of school children had the school board compel [him] to be examined for leprosy because they knew his mother had it, and they found him to have more germs than any one here. What good was isolation for him? Another case, a man from [town is indecipherable] took his daughter to Dr. Deyer (sic)* [Dr. Isadore Dyer, Tulane dermatologist and the man responsible for the Lepers Home and early treatment for leprosy patients in Louisiana] *to be examined and he diagnosed leprosy. The man at once brought her here to protect the other children. This girl was here 15 years refusing her people to visit her to*

*protect them when her father and the other sister had to come here
with leprosy also. A lady cousin of theirs never would associate with
them because she knew of this case and did not want to expose herself
to it so as to protect her self and children, with the results that 8 years
after the first girl came she herself came to find out that she had it
and had to come here. I could relate many more such stories including
mine but much to my sorrow you know it too well. And I hope that I
have been sufficiently punished for such neglect of duty that our kids
will not have to suffer the same results and that you may be spared
from this for your actions towards me.*

[EDMOND CITES INTERNATIONAL MEDICAL EVIDENCE
FOR HIS ARGUMENTS] *I have already recalled Dr. S.[Sabatier]
and Dr. R. [Roussell] statement and will now give you a few others,
which are quoted from a book on leprosy by Sir Leonard Rogers; Text
Book "Pathogenic Microorganisms by Park and Williams, N.Y.;
and from Senate Report # 300 of the 1ˢᵗ session of the 84ᵗʰ congress
when they were trying to pass bill for this National Leprosarium.
"Numerous inoculation experiments have been made on animals
with portions of leprous tubercles, but there is no conclusive evidence
that leprosy can be transmitted to the lower animals by inoculations.
The inference that this bacillus bears an etiological relationship
to the disease with which it is associated is based chiefly upon the
demonstration of its constant presence in leprous tissues. (Because I
handle lots of money does it mean that I am rich: EGL) Although
many attempts have been made to infect healthy individuals with
material containing the bacillus of leprosy the results are not conclusive. Even the experiments made by Arning, who successfully
infected a condemned criminal in the Sandwich Islands with fresh
leprous tubercles, and which have been regarded as positive evidence
of the transmutability of the disease in this way, are by no means
conclusive, for according to Swift, the man had other opportunities
for becoming infected. The negative result, together with the fact that
infection does not more frequently occur in persons exposed to the disease, may possibly be explained by the assumption that the bacilli
contained in the tuberculous tissues are mostly dead, or much more
probably that an individual susceptibility to the disease is requisite*

for its production." P&W in Path. Micro-org. Patient with tuber-
culosis travels on the public carriers, he goes to different resorts and
places where he may be cared for in sanatoria; while on the other
hand, there are few states that do not discriminate against the "lep-
er." (This is the reason for Nat'l Leprosarium. EGL) He (meaning
the "leper") is discriminated against in all public places, to the end
that he becomes an outcast and an object of horror in spite of the fact
that the danger of [contagion] from him is about 1 to 100 as compared
with the tubercular patient. (Dr. Deyer sic) (I have always contend-
ed that. EGL). "Of course there are great many people who are "lep-
ers" who would hardly need to be admitted to such an institution.
These persons are not dangerous of themselves at their own homes. It
would be ridiculous to suppose that every one of the "lepers" would
be better off in the leprosarium than he would be in his own home."
Dr. Rucker, Assist. Surg. Gen. U.S. Pub Health services, Div. of
interstate quarantine. (Dr. Deyer and Dr. Rucher's statements are
taken from the Senate Report.)

"In the first place, most married persons have passed the most
susceptible age and rapidly reach the period of slight susceptibility,
which Leloir says begins to decrease after the age of 20, thus account-
ing for the infrequency of conjugal infection. Munro states that after
the age of 30 years [Claire would be 31 in August of 1928] *the ten-*
dency to be attacked is almost nil"------ "and recorded the case of
a woman in Hawaii escaping the disease in spite of having had 3
'leper' husbands." They report having found germs in "one positive
case in a young virgin with an intact hymen." "A number of attempts
to infect healthy persons by experimentally inoculating them with
fresh lepra bacilli containing material have completely failed, with
the doubtful exception of Arning's case of a convict in Hawaii, who
may have contracted his subsequently developing disease from two
near "leper" relatives. This negative evidence, however, loses much
of its value on account of all the experiments having been carried out
on adults who had passed the most susceptible age period; none of
the ten persons inoculated by Prefeta was under 25." "In many parts
of the world, compulsion has been used to destroy or isolate them
[infected people], but only when they have already infected others
while in the earlier stages of the disease." Many authorities claim

to have successfully cultivated the lepra bacilli, others claim such as impossible and here is the conclusion of Rogers "that the bacillus has never actually been cultivated outside of the human body, and that all the organisms described are contaminations." Fraser and Fletcher sum up their thorough investigation, in which they used the methods of Clegg, Rost, Williams, Duval, and Bayon, without positive results: "Material for purposes of cultivation of various media has now been obtained from 32 non—ulcerating nodular case of leprosy (my type) and 373 inoculations made on the various culture media. It is curious, in view of the findings of other investigators that we have consistently failed to obtain a culture of the leprae bacillus." "In many cases the disease appears to last for many years without the patient ever being conscious of its existence, and then to disappear," "For we hold, as we have argued above, that the mere conveyance of lepra bacilli into the body is not sufficient to bring about the disease; the soil must in some way or other be prepared, so as to enable the disease germs to grow." "The onset of leprosy being as a rule painless and the disease resembling as it does trivial complaints such as ringworms, the patient often neglects to seek early medical advice" (I say, even the one [who] knows he has it fails to seek medical advice so as not to be isolated hence, isolation is really a cause of continuation of the disease. EGL) Leprous patches increase in size much more slowly than those of tinea circinate (Ringworm). Moreover, the almost invariably itching of ringworm is almost always absent in leprosy, or at least in any leprous patches that could be mistaken for ringworm." (All these statements following Dr. Ruckers are quoted from Roger and Muir's book on Leprosy.) I enclose copies of clippings from recent newspapers to one of which I have added a few remarks for your benefit.

[THE TRAGEDY OF SOME PATIENTS]   *Now to corroborate some of these above statements, I will have to tell you a few things that can't be made public but they are nevertheless facts learned here. The proofs of Dr. Dyers statement and reason that he knew as much about leprosy as he did and that he was not scared of it is that he treated and "cured" his wife without sending her here. That is between you and I and the gate post. Some fellows in my locality whom I often wondered how they knew so much about leprosy, since I am here I have found out that their family had very close connections in here, and you know them very well and they are of prominence in N.O. and this state. The more I learn the more that I realize that "What one does not know does not hurt" All my life I lived a clean life fearing dangerous disease and look the number of packages I have had handed to me. One girl here has always been very careful, never did this or that, never slept with any of her brother or sisters, always insisted on having her personal linens, dishes, silverware, and that all these be kept separate from the rest and no one but her has the disease in her family and I would not doubt that she was suspicious because of my case and on examination [found] her to be positive. In my last letter I told you that unless you treated me differently I would not go back home even with a discharge and you have not even replied although it is since the 1ˢᵗ of April, about, besides not having consented to what I asked. Now I will tell you why. Since I have found out just how much you fear this disease I consider that discharges are of no value. For I have seen 16 patients discharged since I am here and I would not change place with more than two of them. One of these two in my estimation was a mistaken diagnosis and the other was in just as good a shape when she came in as when she went out, after being here 7 or eight years. The others all looked much worse than I, as standing together, a well employee, a patient with 14 good tests, and I and we asked a visiting doctor to pick out the patients. He picked me out as the well man, the discharged patient as a "good" case and the employee in a hell of shape. Well, the employee is in a hell of a shape as he has t.b. Others went out of here and on trying to get treatment for other troubles outside, were diagnosed as "lepers" by the examining physicians. Many patients now getting good tests take almost one hour every day to be bandaged. One man stayed in the hospital for 18 months gradually getting worse and he had 12 or 14 good tests when he died. One lady was here 15 years trying hard to get cured and finally she did get one but on finding out that her children did not want her, discharged or not, after always pretending all the time to be anxious to have her back, figuring, I guess, that she would never get one, it was such a shock to her that she died 15 days after the granting of her papers, of a Broken-heart, as recorded here.*

And the worst of all is one discharged man here was offered a job in the laboratory and he was anxious to keep on this job until he finished his studies but he would not be permitted to live on the personnel side with the well people but he would have had to be isolated like the rest of the patients so he declined the position. It is the thought of all these things and the realization of how the public does not care to have us out of here, whether parolees or absconders that all but runs us nuts.

[EDMOND'S DILEMMA]   *But how can the public be blamed for being afraid of cases which they think are of recent date and have no special love or duty towards the afflicted person, when the love and duty of our dear ones cannot prevent them from being scared and really shun us in spite of the fact that they most of the time have been in close contact for 10 years or more. Take my case for instance, all the public think that my case developed while I was sick at home, but I do not think they would be scared if they knew that I had it for 22 years or more and see me in better physical condition now than I ever have been. Claire I stood everything from the day I found out I had this to the time that the Doctor offered me an "equal chance" of getting out of here, thinking that you loved me; but when you refused to do the very least once a month telling me to get my loving among my kind, well I knew then that you did not love me for as I have already told you "Love knows no fear" as proven by some of the wives that visit here. (You will say that it is their ignorance that causes them to be so careless and take chances. Well I wish to God I had married some one that ignorant.) From that day on it has never worried me in the least whether I get a discharge or not. You told me that my having this was the Lord's will and I should bear my cross accordingly, having faith in and praying to the Lord would cure me. It is the Lord's will that I have leprosy but it is your selfish prejudiced will that makes me feel the pain of this "living death," for one visit a month from you would make me forget all and I would feel as if I am at any other place for treatment and fit to be with you and the kids should I ever get paroled but as it is I regard myself as cast away rubbish and you know that it is hard to pull rubbish out of a trash can and make it be something again. So far as your faith and prayers they are, like the rest of the public's, all one sided. When you* can make me understand why "faith and prayers" can't prevent you from catching leprosy by just coming to me once or twice a month, far easier than it can cure me, especially when you take all the foregoing statements in consideration; then I will believe in faith and prayers: and if after you read this you can decide that it is really not the danger that you think it is and come to see me and act differently to what you have, I will then try again to get a parole even though I do not think there is any such thing as a cure as Dr. Heiser or Dean has said "It is impossible to prove the negative of leprosy."

If you will not, don't ever reproach me for anything I may do in the future. Now don't start by telling me about "vowed duties and for the kids sake," that I should do this and that, for I know all that, but the duties and the kids are not only mine. I am standing by my duties and the kids when I stay here but you are not when you refuse to come to see me as I have requested for as I have always said a monthly visit to me as promised in that letter, as per the clipping that I sent you in my last letter, would be more of a cure to me than all the oil [chaulmoogra] that I drink and have shot into me. And I can prove this by Skipper's case who had been getting in worse shape for six years and last summer his wife came here for 3 weeks and treated him and us just the same as if she was a patient herself from that time on Skipper started to get better and when his test came up in Feb. it was good and he now has four good ones. That is the kind of a wife the patients need and the kind that I thought I had but much to my sorrow I have found out different. "A case is recorded where one woman had three 'leper'" husbands without contracting the disease" and statistics show that only about 2 to 5 of cases may arise from marriage, this last fact is enough to keep one from getting married to a "leper" but should not be sufficient to cause one to want to be separated especially when you take in consideration that there is no evidence to prove that this small percentage of cases would not have developed the disease whether they married or not. (when you know that these statistics are made up in countries where 2 to 5% of the population develop leprosy.) In the U.S. we know of many wives sticking with their husbands and vice verse, and others marrying a known "leper," even known absconders from here; and no case caused by marriage is recorded. Dr. Denny told a man patient here "that the only way he might infect his wife was if he had a sore or abrasion on a certain place." I have no sore at such a place nor anywhere else but I did have one there when I was home from Camp Pike on a furlough. [Edmond and Claire had been married by that time.] You once said, "If it was not for the kids you would live with me anywhere" and like a dam fool I believed it but you did not mean it for if you had meant it you would not fear visiting me here once a month, and how would you feel if the Lord would take our kids away so that they would not be in your way sticking by me.

You have said that it is better for me to be here for the protection of the kids and all evidence shows that kids are susceptible to the disease, and maybe, therefore, it is best for me to be here; but how will you reconcile this statement when you consider that you told me personally and that is if you, your mother or brother were to develop it you all would "certainly not come here." Why would you not be equally as afraid of your case as you have been of me? Because as I have said, "Real love fears nothing." That is another statement that has hurt me beyond words. I would not advise you to come here if you were to get it and you agree that you would stay home then why refuse me that little happiness that I ask under the pretext of wanting to protect the kids. Look what happened to me by protecting them before I knew I had this, and had it all the time. The more I staid home the more I exposed them. And after I found out that I had it, I staid home with all belief that there was no danger and really feel still that there was none, but since I know how you feel, it makes me feel like a low down no count curr.

The enclosed copy tells of practically all conditions that one connected with leprosy should be on the look out for. If everybody having any of these conditions were examined for leprosy, first, whether they [were] related to or been in contact with a "leper" or not; not only tested at the 1st attack but at every repeated attack, they would find so many "lepers" in the world that we could not be isolated.

[THERE ARE OTHER SYMPTOMS] Two other conditions that I did not mention are Nasal Catarrh, and Red Ears (Like I always had). Every patients [who] are suffering or have suffered from some nasal trouble some only thought to have been "head colds," as often

*I remember having. And here are some of the findings on this. "Lie I
Norway found 92 and Hellman [or Wellman, author—both names
are associated with leprosy in the early part of the century] in Hawaii
90% in nodular types, 66% in mixed types and 46% in nerve types;
to have positive results from nasal mucus." "Thiroux examined 200
cases and found bacilli in 90% of cases" "Kitasato in Japan examined
the nasal mucus of 68 healthy persons, the issue of "lepers" or [those]
living with them, and in 8 found very numerous bacilli in the epithe-
lial cells. He thinks this is the initial stage of leprosy." (This corroborates my theory on the infection of leprosy EGL) "The fact, however,
that on careful scraping of the nasal mucus membrane, bacilli are not
found, does not exclude a nasal infection or a nasal path of entry of the
bacilli. Just as in skin lesions we have superficially anesthetic patches
in which no bacilli can be found, and also non-anesthetic patches in
which bacilli are found in large numbers (that is what makes it so hard
to make a positive diagnosis of this) so in the nasal mucous membrane
we often find a dry form of rhinitis in early leprosy, but examination of
smears, made from scraping of its surface, fail to show any 'lepra' bacilli. Such patients mention the absence of nasal catarrh, and we have
found this symptom is not infrequently a forerunner of the more appar-
ent initial signs of leprosy." (From R&M's book on Lep.) Now as to
the red ears, you remember mine. Well one patient here told me that
when he was but 4 or 5 years he remembers his mother always looking
at him and saying "I dread to see your ears that red most of the time"
and later on when he was diagnosed as a "leper" she told him that that
is what she had dread for all those years. For instance in my case, if the
ulcer I had on my leg when I was about 10 years old, had been examined for leprosy they very likely would have found me to be one then
and [I] could have been treated for this without being isolated and not
even told about it as it being leprosy but instructed to take precautions
as for T.B. and it would have been sufficient for everybody's protection;
instead of it being said to be a "nee de gaipe" (Wasp's nest) (Mama
would no doubt remember it) and my going 20 years without treatment
or any precautions. After this 20 years of unknowingly exposing the
public and finding out at 30 years old made my case dangerous and
I can't be treated as an ordinary man even though I feel better today,
physically, than I have for the past 16 years.*

[THE INJUSTICE TO LEPROSY PATIENTS]   *Speaking of T.B.,
it reminds me of it and Syphilis. It makes me mad when I think about
them, especially syphilis who medical science let them run wild even
though they can swear that it is infectious by contact and that a non-
syphilitic person can carry the germ from a lesion of the infected person to an innocent person. Syphillis Innocentium (very likely the kind
I had if not inherited from back generations) but they cannot swear
that leprosy is infectious they know that a healthy person cannot carry
it from a "leper" to another healthy person, and they cannot prove
or swear that leprous infected material inoculated in a well person
will develop leprosy, as per statement of Dr. Sabatier; statement of
Dr. Rogers, stated above, that "that conveyance of bacilli is not sufficient to bring about the disease." Dr. Barentine told Skipper's wife
last year, "They say he has leprosy but I could not swear to it." The
state of Florida isolated 15 or 20 cases of leprosy here and treats about
4,000 cases of syphilis every month, at home, as per their State Board
of Health Bulletin every month. Still they the medical science isolate "lepers," but guess they are forced to do it on account of public
prejudiced opinion, and they, nor the public, can't be blamed much
when relatives of patients will go so far as requesting that patients be
locked up in jail to prevent their absconding, or their being brought
back by the parents when they abscond. I get to be a ravin maniac,
almost, when I think that we are not given "equal chances." Take
for instance, syphilitic child or children, from syphilitic parents, not
infected or not known to be infected are permitted to attend school.
Teachers with T.B. teach children at a highly susceptible age, both are
mingling with and exposing healthy children. I don't mean that those
children and teachers should be deprived of their school and their work
but I do contend that we should be given an equal chance, for if I was
to go home to-day my kids would be taken away from school for the
protection of other children even though it is known that a third person cannot carry it, and remember that syphilis is worse than leprosy.
Syphilis is the most insidious and horrible of all known diseases.—
"Instead of being easily destroyed it is gradually spreading throughout the world, steadily tainting the blood and undermining the vital-
ity of human race"—Once introduced into the system—the victim
can never feel sure that he is full rid of its poison." (Dr. Perry)*

[LET ME GET THIS OFF MY CHEST] *You once said that if it was not for the kids you would give me an equal chance, that is, let me leave here and go someplace, with me, where we were not known, if you had meant this you would compromise this now, to just coming one or two days per month and if you can't make two trips per month you could stay two days on one trip as you can now stop at some very nice (white) people's house, but you won't give me this chance even though that you were in close contact with me a "leper" for about 10 years, seven of which were spent without any precautions when we did not know that I had this. And if you had known that Norbert had leprosy before we married and that his case had not been caught in the army as we thought you would not have married me, just because I was his brother. Why Claude [Claire's brother] and your mother would not even have allowed me to visit you. But still it was alright for Claude to court Liz [Liz was Claude's fiancée who died of tuberculosis] (I hate talk about her and may God bless her, but all this has hurt me too much and whilst I am at it I want to get it all off of my chest) and if she had lived he no doubt would have married her, and as I already told you, you would have been her nurse in later years regardless of how much it exposed our kids. I do not mean that Claude should not have courted her for I admire and glorify in a man who courts and marries the one he loves regardless of physical or financial condition nor do I mean that she should not have been nursed by a well person, be it you or any one else for we must all help others for we know not what may some day come to us; but I do claim that we should be given some benefit of the doubt treated like they are instead of being dis-criminated against as we are.*

Claire, I think that when you wrote that letter telling me that you were coming as per the clipping I mailed you in my letter April 1st, about that you had really intended coming but that some person or per-sons scared you and advised you not to come. I don't know, and don't care to know, who they are but you can put it down and remember it when it happens, that whoever it is that did, will suffer before they die, if they have not already suffered, as much or more than I have, not necessarily with leprosy for there are lot of things worse than having leprosy. Now, understand well, I have wished no one any harm at all, but one cannot do a "leper" an injustice and get by with it.

[THE KIDS AND I SUFFER]   *I once said that the kids would grow up to be more afraid of me than you are and good God knows that you are afraid enough; but you said they would be brought up differently. How could they be different?* [Surprisingly, my mother and uncle did not share my grandmother's fear of the disease that claimed their father nor did they communicate fear to any of us. My mother told me that in the 1940s when she and her brother would visit their aunt and uncle in Carville, my grandmother would have a bottle of rubbing alcohol on the table for them to use when they returned. My mother finally said, "Mamma, we are not going to keep doing this."] *When after you having lived with me as you did for years and you have the dreadful fear that you have, which they will understand when they reach the age of better understanding, they naturally will be more afraid as they will figure that they have practically never been exposed to it. I have learned too much since I am here, a "leper" never had a chance. First, the children are babies and highly susceptible; second, they have to be allowed to go through school; third, their social career and standing must be considered; fourth, their political or commercial affairs cannot be sacrificed; and last but not least, the in-laws object, if they don't, grandchildren now arrive on the scene and have to be protected like the first generation and the same routine is started over. One man here lived through this ordeal with his children telling him, and he believing them, that they wanted him back thinking, I guess, that he could not get away; so one day he packed up and went. Well, two or three weeks later his children brought him back, and it grieved him so that he shortly after died of nothing but a broken heart. Other similar cases could be cited. It's hell; the law and you want me here, and I had agreed to stay but then you refuse to compromise by coming as I asked. You won't bring the kids to see me here and won't let me go home to see them.* [Because children were highly susceptible to leprosy, they were not allowed as visitors at the hospital. However, the laws were broken at times and children did come to visit parents or siblings. At other times, patients escaped through the hole in the fence to visit family outside of the institution. My grandmother strictly adhered to the laws and I never got the sense that my mother or her brother even knew they could have visited their father.] *Gee, Claire that surely always drives back to my memories that heart rendering statement that you made to me one day "they are my children and I'll etc" I've tried to forget it but it always comes back. Why Claire, if it was not for the letter of acknowledgement that I get from them when I send something, I would think that they had forgotten about me. You may not realize it but I have been here nearly 4 years and never have they (if they do you never told me) shown any anxiety about me such as children of their age would; such as asking "How is my Daddy?" "When is my Daddy coming home?" etc. Of course it is hard to think that Daddy never will be well and be home to them, as any other daddy would be; but they do not know this and it would sound good to know that they are interested. Only one time did one of them inquire "How is my Daddy" but that was a few days after one of your visits here at which time I had mentioned this same matter to you.*

[THIS DISEASE IS NOT LIKE OTHERS] *Coming back to discharges, I overlooked to mention the fact that some of them relapse and come back. Some lady discharged since I am here I understand she is having trouble and may have to come back. Another one I heard had failed to show up for her semi-annual test. This all indicates that others have similar faith but from their first experience won't come back. The general public does not know this fact but it is so. Most all other diseases relapse also and this should make no difference but our disease is never considered like others. And that is why a discharge does not worry me for if I would ever get one I never would want to come back here. Knowing how it can come back and how you dread this I would always be worried about it coming back and to have to come here again. If you would act as I asked you for two years it would encourage me to get well, as shown you about Skipper's case, for I'd know in the event that I did get a discharge you would not be afraid of me if I was unfortunate enough to have it come back on me again and I would not have to worry about returning here unless circumstances forced me, and if I had to return I would know that you would still treat me as I wish.*

[JUST HOW MUCH THIS HURTS]   *Claire, you advised me not to run away from here, declined to assist me to get out of here on that Doctor's plan, and last, but not least, refused to come to me once per month as I tried to compromise, it hurt so much that I tried to disappear but failed as I have already told you. To give you an idea of just how much it did hurt I will say that it hurt me more than if I, on returning from some of my salesman's trip, had found you with another man and you know that would have hurt me some. Just think how you would have felt if you had found me making love to a stenographer and double that heartache and you will have a slight idea of how I felt. But that may not amount to much since you can keep away from me as you do. Therefore, I will put it another way. Rather than have this and be treated as I am, I would prefer to be blind at home with you to love and care for me.*

Speaking of blindness it reminds me of the time that I told you, one day when you were here, how I dreaded the thought of becoming blind or developing T.B. in this place and now that I know how possible it is for me to get one if not both afflictions with hardly no prophylactic treatment in view it almost runs me nuts when I think of it especially that I now know that you would not do as you promised. "Don't worry if you do become either, I will go with you anywhere that I can be with you and take care of you." And now that I also know how you feel about this disease, I could not permit you to do so and feel right conscientiously, about it. Of course, you said "It is not necessary to try to cross a bridge before we get to it." These sad facts are unfortunately our lot and the sooner they are faced the more complications may be avoided for the future.

[COMPULSORY ISOLATION IS USELESS]   *To corroborate the fact that, the grievance that I have against medical science on account of their permitting compulsory isolation, which I contend is an injustice to the "lepers," I quote a statement that I read this morning. It is from a circular report reprinted from "The Practitioner" April, 1928, issue. It goes along and compares the effectiveness of voluntary hospitalization against the impossible complete compulsory segregation and suggests new plans, concluding as follows: "This economic and effective plan will entirely replace compulsory isolation and* *perhaps the <u>greatest remaining reproach</u> (my underscore EGL.) to scientific medicine will disappear."*

And this statement is made by none other than Sir Leonard Rogers, the world's greatest renowned Leprologist, of England. England in India has over one million recorded cases and he, Rogers says there is probably more than 3 times that many actual cases which would be about twenty times more than there is under segregation. And I think if the truth was known here the proportion of isolation cases and cases at large would be about the same or more.

The above mentioned circular is sent to Doctors, so I am writing to Dr. Carstens to try to procure me a copy of same. Will have him let you read it before mailing it to me, but it will take some time as it is printed in London and don't know where to get from any U.S. Publisher.

This famous doctor also states and recommends the following "As leprosy is so frequently a house infection with an incubation period commonly extending from one to five years, when a new case of leprosy is found everyone living in the same house, including both relatives and domestics, should at once be examined for early signs of the disease, and this should be repeated every three or six months for five years, if possible to enable all the infections arising from the first case to be detected and cured while in the early amenable stages. By this means one focus of infection will be eradicated, and a definite step taken towards preventing the spread of leprosy and reducing the incidence of the disease." This you refuse to do and give for your reason that "It may be best not to know." Why have you changed your view point on this? You use to think that it was best to know when my case was in doubt and even though Dr. Sabatier stated that my case was not leprosy, you and the others thought it advisable and best for me to consult a specialist and bacteriologist that we should know positively what it was. Since you see danger of contagion for you and the kids in only one or two days visit to me per month, it is obvious that the several years that I unknowingly exposed you all was far more dangerous and enough so to make observations, as recommended above, necessary. I am here, and willing to stay here to protect the kids (protection to you now seems unnecessary as per Roger's Books states and mentioned above. Also Dr. Wooley's statement to me, that "after 25 it was hardly possible to contract leprosy" and in all his practice he had never seen a single case who had not had contact prior to the age of thirty) but where is the protection if you, unbeknown to yourself are infected for you are with them far more than I ever was or will be. Also if you are already infected what is the use of your being afraid of me. If you were not infected, but unfortunately, one or both kids, who according to medical science are highly susceptible, should have been infected; what is the use of my isolation or your fears? Roger's states "One even, when he suspects what his ailment may be, is afraid lest he should lose his employment keeps his disease a secret till it can no longer be hid. In this way, not only does the patient prejudice what chance he has of recovery, but in many cases he exposes those who come in contact with him"

"Although tuberculosis is far more easily transmitted than leprosy, the known sufferer from pulmonary tubercle is allowed to mix in society while the known "leper" is shunned. This is largely a survival of the aboriginal superstition that leprosy is in some way or other a sign of the special displeasure of the gods. But it is unreasoned fear on the part of the general public which inspires fear in the mind of the patient and keeps him back from presenting himself to the medical practitioner for early diagnosis and treatment"

[YOU MAY HAVE SOME SYMPTOMS]   *You could get Dr. Johns to make these periodical examinations of you and the kids since he did not report me [I] don't see why he would report any of you all, if unfortunately it did show up. As Dr. Johns told me, "As hard as it is, it is best for one to know." Of course, you say that you all have no signs of the disease and never had it in any ancestors. I neither know of any ancestry for my case but on this point our kids certainly have. Now as to manifestations and characteristics of the disease you may have one of the many, as named on the enclosed copy of clippings, even though the doctor diagnoses it as positively something else. As my case, Dr. S[abatier] said that it was not leprosy even though he knew that Norbert had it and the N.O. Dr. did not recognize it, at first, taking it for Erythema Nodosum but on bacterial examination it was proven to be this. Dr. S., at about the time that it was not known what I had, examined an erythematous patch on your back and diagnosed it as ringworm. I remember this spot and it is exactly similar to many that I have seen here. I once asked you, when you were here, about it and you replied that it had healed, but you would not show me that it was, when I asked you to show me. I don't want to say that this spot was really a leprosy lesion but it would be best to know, for it is said that in many instances when the primary lesion was recognized and excised, the disease disappeared never to return. Besides this spot you have funny looking toes which you claim comes from tight shoes and I hope it is but remember that such toes are very characteristic of this disease. Seems to me that I also remember hearing you say that your skin had a "muddy" appearance no matter how much you washed it and this is about the only sign that I have left on my lower limbs and forearms. Of course you will say that you never had other symptoms to indicate this, but don't forget this "In many cases the disease appears to last for many years without the patient ever being conscious of its existence and then to disappear" I am not telling you all this because I wish you to find any of these signs but so that you will know them and be able to profit by my experience, for if you will recall that was one of my reasons for coming here—to find out just what this was and how it worked for our future information—so since these are facts we have to face them as hard as they may seem. So for God's sake if you or either of the kids have or in the future get any signs pointed out in this letter don't take any chances with any doctor but have examinations made by a skin specialist and Bacteriologist, giving them the information that they have been in contact with leprosy. Now as to ancestry, as said before, none of mine have nor have had it, as much as we know; but many have some or have had some of disease mentioned, all of which may come from one of two conditions which in my estimation has existed for three generations and on which I base my theory that leprosy comes from something else and not the Bacillis Leprea; this bacilli being caused by some bodily condition instead of the condition being caused by the bacilli. Now as to your ancestors, I leave it to you to judge whether they had any such similar troubles or not as you know better than I do.*

[REACTIONS OF LEPROSY PATIENTS TO TREATMENTS]
Every person who is known to be affected with leprosy, when taking potas. Iodide gets a reaction, some more violent than others according to their sensitiveness or the dose taken, just like when I take a few small doses, I get a headache, cold in the head, itch, new tubercles and the old ones are aggravated; if I still persist taking it I get nauseated and feverish, and nerve pains and this is because I have leprosy. "Some observers have found that the administration of potassium iodide facilitates the finding of lepra bacilli in the nasal mucus *when given an hour before the examination is made." (R. 16) When an outsider takes potassium iodide and gets practically the same results he has not leprosy, but iodium, "A term applied to the condition produced by the* prolonged *use of iodine and its compounds. It is characterized by violent coryza, headache, a metallic taste in the mouth, (I remember a bad taste too but not just what it tasted like) increased salivary secretion, (Guess I would get this also if I had taken it long enough for slight facial paralysis frequently causes "slobbering") gastric irritation, an acne rash. The incorporation of tr. Belladonna (Min 5) with each dose of iodide will generally prevent the disagreeable catarrhal symptoms." (Scott's Cyclop. 488) You remember Dr. S[abatier] gave me a lotion of Soda hyposalphite, Rx 274254, when he prescribed potas. Iod. Rx 278919, after having first tried Fowler's Sol. Rx 278255 with same lotion for any rash following. Who knows that if these people suffering from "iodium" were tested would not prove to be in the very incipient state of leprosy, or maybe syphilis since potass. Iod. is used for treatment in both, as "Danielsson in 1886 used potassium iodide extensively in the treatment and diagnosis of the disease. Wolffe, also considered it to be of diagnostic value, as he observed febrile reactions, with the appearance of lepra bacilli in the blood, the appearance of old nodules and the appearance of new ones, during its use. Other observers found increased discharge of lepra bacilli from the nose after its administration, of diagnostic value." "All experiences have shown the great value of iodides in influencing the disappearance of syphilitic lesions." And I read somewhere that iodide would often cause a negative Wasserman to become positive but I can't locate it to quote the real words. I contend that large percentage of old uncured cases of syphilis is an unrecognized case of leprosy,*

combined with it; and many or most of the bad cases of leprosy has
syphilis as a concomitant disease, for as a rule, the worse the condi-
tion of a "leper" the higher the "plus Wasserman." It is also known
that leprosy very rarely causes death but syphilis often does, as I read
a statement sometimes back that 85% of all heart failure could be di-
rectly traced to syphilis. Still a "leper" will not be given any chances.

[In his letter, Edmond made a note that this next paragraph was
for page seven. It is not clear to me where these lines belonged on
page seven of the original, so they are left here despite Edmond's
note that they belong elsewhere.]

"the earlier the treatment the better. Patients may be expected to
make better progress when they are able to continue their daily work.
If an early diagnosis is made and treatment begun at once, there can
be no objection in the majority of cases to the patient continuing his
work."

[I WON'T RETURN HOME EVEN WITH A DISCHARGE]   *When*
I told you in my last letter, that if you did not treat me differently I
would not go home discharged or not, it no doubt made you angry and
you must say that it is unreasonable. Well you won't see me without
a discharge and since I know of the fear that you have I don't think it
right and would not feel right for the following facts. "The term ab-
solute cure should be reserved for those who have passed through the
third stage and have a high degree of immunity. It will be realized
that without this immunity in a disease in which the germs can lie
latent for over twenty years and then light up and produce leprosy in
an acute form, it is impossible to prophecy that circumstances will not
occur in which some few lepra bacilli, still hiding among the tissues
of the body will again produce the disease in a patient who formerly
suffered and is now apparently cured."

"The fact that smears from the deeper organs in ten out of eleven
cases on the negative list were found bacteriologically positive at au-
topsy, and that in nine out of 53 cases smears of material aspirated
from the femoral lymph nodes were positive, Pineda says is in accord
with the generally recognized fact 'lepers' are not necessarily bacil-
lus-free when they become negative by ordinary methods of examina-
tion. The skin and, apparently the spleen and liver become negative

comparatively early, while other sites, (especially the nerves, lymph nodes and testes) the infection tends to persist for a relatively long time. It is particularly of interest that the patients examined by aspiration were nearing the end of the required two year negative period." Therefore, unless that you can show that you are willing to treat me right as I am (for all patients and everybody remark how much better I look than those on negative test and cannot understand why I am still positive), I can't see that a discharge will make me much safer.

[I DON'T WANT TO DISAPPEAR]   *Sometimes back when I told you that you were not treating me right, you said you were doing the best you could and that your road was as hard for you as mine was for me but I told you it was not and that you may be sorry someday but then it would be too late. Claire you think you are unhappy now, but you have kids, your home, your daily work, and your mother; in fact you have all that you have ever had except me. Your mother is there to help you now but remember she is not immortal although she may outlive me. Claire just stop and think how you refused me the little happiness that I asked of you even after placing all common-sense facts before you and warning you that things that had to be would happen whether I staid in isolation or not and whether you visited me or not. Of course I hope that such will never happen but just suppose, for a moment, that in years to come these facts and warnings would come true, how would you regret those years of heartache unnecessarily caused to us both during these years should I still be living; and the sad reproaches you would make yourself if it should happen after I am dead and gone and not there to help and console you. Why Claire, your road of present sadness would be like a road of roses as compared to the road of sorrow you would then have. It is this thought—of how you and the kids may need me in the future—and the love that I have had for "home" that has kept me so far from disappearing. However, on account of the way you are acting towards me, this thought is almost gone and the love of home has gradually died and is practically dead and unless you can do something to revive it in the very near future, I will not be here very much longer. Please do not let it die for there is nothing deader than a dead love.*

[SOME OTHER FACTS ABOUT THIS DISEASE] *There is so much to be said about the different symptoms of this disease that when you write about them there is always some that are overlooked. Therefore, coming back to the matter of disease being often taken for other troubles, one that I forgot to mention is that "Many patients here have had spots to come and go that were always diagnosed as simply 'liver spots' but later proved to be leprosy." Leprosy has a tendency of self-healing, and may or may not return. Did the removing of your tooth stop your ear-ache. I have had ear ache for three years, and had a spell for the last ten days but it is better to-day as it is getting warmer. I remember pains in my ears long before I knew I had this, not continuous but frequently.*

Now another thing that gets me about this as compared to syphilis is that "Syphilis is a serious disease, paradoxical as it may seem, because its course is so indolent. It is in this respect like tuberculosis and leprosy." "We cannot protect the healthy against infection of syphilis by isolation as can be done with acute infectious diseases which run a short time. The period of infectiousness in syphilis is much longer, and most important of all, the number of syphilitics is so enormous that isolation or quarantine is impossible. Even personal identification and supervision of them indiscriminately by health authorities has been a notorious failure. The reasons for secrecy are so strong, prejudices or feelings about sexual morality are so varied, and motives and sentiments so divided, that laws for reporting syphilis and other venereal disease are not sustained by the public sentiment; and like all other laws, which sentiment is not behind, are ineffective. This, in my opinion, makes laws for the notification of syphilis—with identification of the patients—undesirable." 95% of syphilis cases comes through immorality, in other words one afflicted with it has looked for it, whilst such is not the case in one afflicted with leprosy; but still the laws are—secrecy for syphilis and publicity for leprosy—even though syphilis is far more infectious. Now don't forget what I warned you about Claude's condition that has chased him to N.Y. I know several patients here who have had this very same trouble followed up by syphilis and finally landed here. That is why I told you to tell him to get married and settle down.

Many fellows down home, who now know I have this, if they ever come to find out about it, they will immediately say that they got if from me but if there was any "catching" done, I caught it from them. John Landry is afraid to visit here, and so are the rest of the boys at the store, and they rub with some worse than me two and three times per week if not every day. That is just like the saying about "what one does not know does not hurt."

[YOU AND THE CHILDREN WILL BE TAKEN CARE OF]   *Now as to money matters, you get $100. from the Gov; board from Dum, $25.00 monthly average for N.Y. Life and Pacific Inc., about 15.00 monthly for interest on $250.00 Realty stock, making about $170.00, monthly total. You surely can live on that and as to savings for the kids' future, don't suppose that "Dum" will disinherit them because their father unfortunately was a "leper"; and that will be more than I could give or save for them. The amount I keep here which you say I waste, I spend it by "Making those that are more unfortunate than I, happy" (And believe me there are many such from the financial side especially) and a few little luxuries for myself. Since "Charity covers a multitude of sins" I hope that the little charities that I have done and will try to continue doing will atone, in a way, for the sins I have committed and for those committed in the future. Speaking of "advance" charity, I would have liked you to take Priscilla when she was discharged and I even hinted to you but as you did not notice the hint I said no more about it, because if you had taken her after my asking you to do so and later on with her at home one of the kids should have developed this, the blame would have been placed on her. I do not mean for you to have adopted her but just to give her a home where she could have come to visit her mother frequently. That would have been a nice piece of charity to undertake in asking God a blessing of my cure and deliverance of you and our kids from such fate; and at the same time showing the world that you were not afraid of a discharged "leper." (If she ever had leprosy she surely had less signs than our kids or any that I have ever seen.) Of course, you will say that you could not have taken care of her and our two kids, but what would you have done if I had left you with three kids, you certainly* *would have cared for them so you could have done the same with her especially with what her mother makes here and sends her. I heard yesterday that the people with whom she is living are coming south this summer to visit some relatives and they will take Priscilla along and leave her off here, on their way to Alabama, to spend a few days with her mother.*

Now as to the two insurance policies that are not matured, the one of the Maccabees is alright for it will mature in about ten years but the one of the K. of C. will have to be paid on as long as I live, so it is really not of much value and since I am no more a practical Catholic, not having made my Easter Duties nor do I know when I will feel fit to make them, I am not entitled to membership any more and may not be entitled to benefits, so it would be better for you to get the "cash surrender value" of the policy and obtain a withdrawal card from the order for me.

[THE CHILDREN NEED TO KNOW ABOUT ME WHEN THEY GET OLDER] *Whilst I think of it I want to mention this. If this is to be the last "talk" that we are going to have; remember that it is alright for you to raise the children in ignorance of this disease until they are old enough to understand but then they should be told.* [*In June of 1928 Teenie was nine and Booz was six.*] *And if ever they decide that they want to marry do not let this knowledge keep them from doing so but see to it that the contracting party knows of it also and that he or she taking up this contract with them will be willing to stick by them in the event that this should come to them after marrying as it did me.* [My father spoke to the family doctor, Dr. Flory, before he and my mother were married, and Dr. Flory assured him there was no need to be concerned. When my Uncle Booz was ready to marry he offered his fiancée the same option. She accepted the earlier assurance that Dr. Flory had offered her brother-in-law.] *In the event that this wish of mine is not carried out and in the future this would unfortunately, come to one of them as it did me; I hope, and they will deserve that their partner leave them at once. I don't mean to leave them as you did me but to at once legally annul the marriage.*

[ARE YOU FAITHFUL TO ME OR TO YOUR PRINCIPLES?]
*You once said that you were "Being faithful to me and would love
me a plenty when I would be well; but that will do me about as
much good as if I banked plenty money for you to use when you
are one hundred years old. I have never doubted your faithfulness,
in the least, and know that you will take care of the kids as well
as you can but now lets see if this faithfulness is due to the love
you have for me or just faithfulness to your principles. Supposing,
instead of developing leprosy when I did and having to come here,
that I would have gotten to be a gambler, gone to drinking and coming home drunk and beating you and the kids, you would have left
me—and no one could have blamed you—but you know that you
would not have re-married and would have taken care of the kids
just like the same. Would that have been faithfulness to me or to
your principle. And what good is the love that you will have for me,
when I get well; when under the circumstance you are making me
feel that I never can be sufficiently well to associate with any other
but my kind.*

*You say that any deviation from our agreement may cause chil-
dren to be born. I say that with a little privation and precaution
none would be born and if any were born it would have to be looked
upon as you always say, "As the will of God" and we would not be
a bit more subjected to this than the two we had before I found out
what my ailment was. If you had always been against birth control it would be different but you have always said that you certainly never would have more than 3 or 4 kids; so if you could have
controlled the number then, why could you not do the same now? I
never was for a race suicide, but think that birth control, under some
circumstances, in order. I never had believed in "free love" but I
surely do want more loving than I am getting and if you won't give
me the very least loving, as requested, according to church and state
law; my only recourse is with my kind and according to common-
law, or "companionate way." I used to believe only in legal church
kind but I have come to realize that couples that will stick to each
other "for better or for worse" will do so equally as well under the
"companionate" kind as those married at Solemn Nuptial, even
at two Nuptial ceremonies with both wives living as I know of one*

case; the "until death do us part" really means so little these days that the rituals should be made to read "for better or worse until one of us sees fit to part whether the partner agrees or not." You said that I was unreasonable for "If I consulted anyone they would give you right" but what chance of justice has a "leper" with discriminating, prejudiced public, who besides being prejudice does not know all the forgoing facts which I have told you, all of which you know to be true. You know that I am a "leper" and shun me so to the extent that you think that one visit per month could make you one also; in spite of the fact that you say you "know that the years you lived with me as such has not infected you" even though that these years were at the time of susceptibility. It is these two last facts that make me insistent on your visiting me for it is like Skipper told you his wife had said, "Why should I be afraid of him now when I was with him for the four years or more that he has had it" and Claire these words were not from her lips to cheer him but from her very heart as proved by her visit here last summer. She would like to move to N.O. to visit him every Sunday but is unable to do so on account of a very good position to which she has worked herself up to in the last six years, and you will not even accept an offer made you there. [My grandmother was originally from New Orleans and still had relatives there. It is possible that a relative or acquaintance may have offered her support. One of the most poignant reactions from my mother was when she told me that she thought her father had wanted her mother to live with him in Carville. My mother was in her eighties at the time but her remark had the pain of a child, "But what would she have done with us?"] *That is just like I always said, this is a funny world "When one can she won't and when one can't she wants."*

I could see this separation coming from the first year that I was here but tried not to let myself believe that you would give me up like this and prayed daily, made novenas to nearly every saint on the calendar, went to Communion every month and oftener but you kept drifting further and further away until I got disgusted and resolved that "if the love for me in your heart could not prompt you to stick with me" I certainly was not going to bother the Lord about it anymore. From that day on I have not been able to pray. All I hope for is that "The Lord will have mercy on me a poor sinner."

Claire, I have told you all of the above so that you will know all fact before you say positively and finally that you will not come back to me as I request so that in the future if anything, that I have warned you of, should happen you will not be able to say "You never had told me and if you had, this or that would not have happened."

[I WILL BE LOVED BY MY OWN KIND]   *The forgoing covers all except one subject which I tried hard to avoid so much so that all the women here thought I was woman shy or a woman hater; you continually refused to come like I asked you and told me to get my loving amongst my own kind so the enclosed letter is what this has resulted to. I have had this letter for months but had not mailed it to you in hopes that you would come for Easter Sunday and everything could have been alright and it would have been unnecessary for you to know this, but you still will not come so I hope that this letter will make you realize what a serious mistake you are making. As [I] told you in first part of this letter your actions towards me has gradually and practically killed the love I had for you and home and unless you act differently toward me, I will go to her and as you have said "my kind."* [My grandfather apparently had a relationship with a woman in Carville. They may have shared his cottage. I do not know who the woman was but these comments seem to allude to such a relationship, as do later remarks in this letter. There is allegedly another missing letter to my grandmother in which my grandfather tells her he plans to go to Brazil and to take the children with him. My mother has also said that she thought her father might have lived with someone in Carville and she could not blame him for that.]

You will say that this is terrible, horrible, etc. for a man to make such a statement to his wife but Claire remember that this is not a bit different to, and the result of, your statement to your husband. Claire, now we are even so come to me soon, let's forget this and be happy again like we were in the past. You know real well that a man's greatest craving, from cradle to grave is for "A woman's love and caresses," and even though I am a "leper" I am still human. Men who have their wives, children, home even the very best kind as you were and as happy home as you and the kids made; and their daily works, still they often drift away from all of it, as you often read about on the paper, to be with another woman, so how could I help from it when I am taken from my kids, home, and work, by force and my wife, the last that I had hope in for just some little happiness, has failed me also, at a time of greatest need. It would be hard if this colony would forbid visitors like they do in some others, but it is still harder to think that visitors are allowed at any time and you refuse to come. When I see how one man here treats his wife, he comes to see her two and three time a week and on Sundays also. On Sundays he often drives here early enough to go to church with his wife and spend the whole day with her until eight or nine o'clock that night. Of course she has six good tests but it did not make any difference to him when she was positive; and you were just as scared of me when I had four good tests as you ever were. I see other wives visit their husbands here, especially some husbands that are here because of their dissipation after they know that they had this & knowing that such living was sure to make him worse, still their wives stick to them, but when I think how you shun me after, even though I say it myself, I have been the husband I tried to be to you, it has made me want to be with and have nothing to do with, any one but 'lepers' from now on. And it is up to you to say right now whether this will be or not.

You will say "Please don't do this for the kids' sake." They would be better off if I had died when Booz was six months old; [April 1922, a month before Edmond's first official diagnosis] *for then it would have been best because nobody would have known anything and all would have avoided these heartaches. Now as to "for the kids sake" lets make it 50–50 for their sake for they are not only my kids; I will stay here for their sake until discharged if you will visit me as requested, to help me get well for their sake if not for mine.*

You will say that this girl does not really care for me and that I will come to find out that it was just a passing infatuation. I don't think so and if you do make me leave here and go to her and she does disappoint me it will not be any greater disappointment than I have already had. But I do know that, being my kind, she would not shun me even though I did get in very bad shape again (even though I am in very good shape to-day does not mean what I will look like in the next 3 or 4 years) It is this last thought and the knowledge of how you dreadfully fear this that makes me feel that I am only fit for a

-18-

If this girl was here just to help/me with my theory as she did when she was here, I would take a chance on a certain inoculation and very likely prove what leprosy is caused by. Cant see how my theory, rather "our" theory now, can be far wrong. For two years I've figured on many different ways to show my point but have just thought of a positive way if I am correct. But if I fail I want no one but a leper to nurse me and she is the only qualified registered leper nurse that I know of. I would prefer not trying this outside but guess I will have to if she cannot get back here. So it will mean some more delay.

There is lots of paper talk in Calif. predicting discontinuation of isolation since the publication of Dr. Walker's article, copy of which I enclose herewith, but of what good will that be to me since you have plainly shown me your feelings, and you still refuse to change your attitude, towards me.

If I were dead, no one would think anything if you remarried, so if you still insist that I belong to the "land of the living death", I should be entitled to seek for a little happiness and companionship with a mate among the "unburried deads" like myself.

I leave it to you to decide, and hope, for the best.

Edmond

Final page of Edmond's eighteen-page letter. He gave Claire the freedom to decide their fate. (Landry Letters from Carville; used with permission.)

"leper" partner from now on; and if you keep on treating me as you have in the past, after you read this letter, I will conclude that you think that is what I am only fit for. You don't want me as a "leper" and I feel that I will be one all my life, so if she was still here you would not have to know a thing about this but she has had to leave here and before I disappear from here, to be with my kind, I want to give you a final chance to keep me for yourself "for better or for worse" and on account of my duty and the love that I have had for you, which could be fully revived, I feel sure that I would be happier with you if you would stick to me now. Guess you will say that "one who loves, loves but one." Well that saying is true as far as it goes, and I don't think that there ever was a husband, who loved only one, more than me. But if the one who originated this saying would have been given the chance to finish this true saying it would have ended with "If that one loves him."

I have always told you that I think this is from some heredity but all books contradict this, except lately an article comes out which reads; "Of 104 placenta examined by Pineda, fifty seven were found positive. In 25 cases the organism was also found in the cord blood. In only one case was the organism found in the cord and not in the *placenta. Histologic examination of placenta and cord did not show any pathologic changes attributable to leprosy. Intra-uterine infection in leprosy should be considered in some cases, particularly when the disease develops in early infancy." I say it is latent in infancy, not often recognized in childhood (unless there is known contact) as quoted before that it can exist long before patient is ever conscious of it; and diagnosed later on when aggravated by some secondary infection.*

If this girl was here to help me with my theory as she did when she was here, I would take a chance on a certain inoculation and very likely prove what leprosy is caused by. Can't see how my theory, rather "our" theory now can be far wrong. For two years I've figured on many different ways to show my point but have just thought of a positive way if I am correct. But if I fail I want no one but a "leper" to nurse me and she is the only qualified registered "leper" nurse that I know of. I would prefer not trying this outside but I guess I will have to if she cannot get back here. So it will mean some more delay.

There is lots of paper talk in Calif. Predicting discontinuation of isolation since the publication of Dr. Walker's article, copy of which I enclose herewith, but of what good will that be to me since you have plainly shown me your feelings, and you will refuse to change your attitude, towards me.

If I were dead, no one would think anything if you remarried, so if you still insist that I belong to the "land of the living death," I should be entitled to seek for a little happiness and companionship with a mate among the "unburied deads" like myself.

I leave it to you to decide, and hope, for the best.

Edmond

SOME REFLECTIONS

"I leave it to you to decide and hope for the best."
Close of Edmond's letter to Claire, June 1928

This long, painful letter is clearly my grandfather's cry from the heart. It represents years of pain that have been ignored and now rupture in a plea to be treated as a human being, as the man he is despite his condition. It rambles around its central theme but that theme is clear: "Be with me as the woman I love. Say now if you will be with me." He used multiple strategies to argue his case for acceptance: research from the best leprologists of the time, the personal experience of Carville patients who were visited by spouses and family, and the dire consequences to patients who were rejected. He argues forcefully against the unjust and needless incarceration of leprosy patients while railing that those with far more contagious diseases, syphilis and tuberculosis, had relative freedom. On a personal note, he pleads for acceptance by his wife, contending that he is much less a threat to her now than during all the past years they shared as husband and wife. He pleads for regular conjugal visits from his wife and longs for acknowledgment from his children.

The letter is a painful insight into my grandfather's desperate loneliness, but it is also an indictment of my grandmother, a woman I loved dearly. Paralyzed by fear, she clearly was unable to be the wife my grandfather desired. My grandfather suggested that "perfect love drives out fear," but my grandmother's human love, however true and stalwart it may have been, was not always perfect. Fear triumphed for many years.

I don't know what I would have done if this letter had proved to be evidence of the end of my grandparents' relationship. I came to know and admire my grandfather through his letters, but I knew and loved my grandmother. She was a central figure in my life. Writing about a non-reconciliation would have felt like an invasion of privacy and a betrayal of my grandmother. However, my grandparents were reconciled, slowly. The letter is testimony to a painful period in their lives, but it is also a letter about second chances in a relationship. It is about the incredible courage of my grandfather to express his desires and about the eventual willingness of my grandmother to meet his needs in some way. It is about a love that was not always or ever perfect but was one of reconciliation sought, forgiveness offered, and recriminations left behind. My grandmother had second chances; my grandfather gave her that. The relationship between the two of them redeveloped slowly, painfully, and no doubt with much scar tissue, but they maintained a relationship until my grandfather's death in December 1932.

My grandfather did not leave Carville as he threatened. In August of 1928, only two months after this letter, he acknowledged to his family that things were not yet as he wanted but that he hoped that Claire would visit. On other occasions he mentioned writing to Claire, hearing from her, and receiving visits from her. In 1931, when the *Sixty Six Star* began to be published, visits to Gabe Michael by his wife were mentioned. The letter of June 1928 was not the end of their relationship nor the last time they talked but it was a pivotal letter for both.

My grandfather remained in Carville but did not succumb to the lethargy of the place. He worked for the betterment of the institution, remained involved in the political and social activities of the hospital, still read widely about his condition, and reacted strongly against the injustices he perceived. His letters to his parents after 1928 became shorter and less frequent but he may have written more regularly to his wife once they had effected a reconciliation.

We have less evidence of my grandmother's personal reaction. She did write to him, return to visit him, and she was with him on the day he died, having been called to Carville at his request. This much we know from evidence, but she kept her own story private, gently avoiding our questions and taking to the grave the secrets of her heart.

Edmond's Letters from Carville to Hospital and Government Personnel

DEAR SIR—YOURS TRULY

> *"At your service now or any other time."*
> Gabe Michael to Dr. O. E. Denney, February 1928

We assume today that patients have at least a degree of autonomy concerning their medical conditions, but this was not always the case. In the early 1900s those who were ill submitted themselves to the medical professionals whose training and expertise made them the presumed experts. The role of the sick was to take prescribed treatments and follow doctors' orders. Their stance was what Arthur W. Frank called a "restitution narrative" (76 ff.). Patients were expected to do what they were told and they would recover. Since there was no real cure for leprosy, patients in Carville had a bit more agency in their treatment. They were allowed some freedom in directing their medical care, taking their medicine, and maintaining personal hygiene and a healthy diet. Because they were in a unique medical community different even from other federal sanatoriums, they also had more freedom within the confines of that institution. Edmond's personal research, as well as letters to Dr. Denney, the Veterans Bureau, and other medical personnel indicates that he did manifest autonomy in his life as a patient and member of the Carville community.

The following letters, whether signed Gabe Michael or Edmond Landry, indicate that my grandfather took seriously his own needs as well as those of his family and fellow patients. This last collection includes copies of some letters from Edmond's medical records now in my possession.

Dr. O. E. Denny
Carville, La.

Dear Sir;—
    There will be several matters of importance coming up before the Executive Committee of the What Cheer Club on next Saturday including a conference with Mr. Rummel in regards to his competition. This is to request you to honor us with your presence at that meeting; Saturday 7:30 P.M.

Yours truly

Gabe Michael
Sec & Treas.
W.C.C [What Cheer Club]
Carville La
Feb. 8th 1925

"*Several matters of importance . . .*" Edmond entered Carville in October 1924. By February, he had organized the Patients' Canteen and the "What Cheer Club," of which he was secretary and treasurer.

"*Honor us with your presence . . .*" The military were clearly in charge of the hospital but also clearly separated from the patients. I don't know if this request was a courtesy to Dr. Denney or an expectation by the MOC that he would be kept apprised of the club's activities. I also do not know if he actually attended the meeting.

Dr. O. E. Denny
Carville, La

Dear Sir:—As per instructions from Executive Committee of the
What Cheer Club, I enclose herewith a copy of complaints on meals
[those complaints are not available in my grandfather's collection].
Desire to remind you of the following matters discussed.
Moving of Tower
15 Loads of Sand for Base Ball Diamond
Additional Park Benches
Moving Picture Machine needing attention.

Yours truly,
Gabe Michael

Sec. & Treas.
W.C.C.
Carville, La.

Feb. 23, 1925

"*Matters discussed.*" This brief note is informative about patient life at
Carville. The patients felt empowered to exercise grievances about meals
and requests for recreational equipment. The tower might have been the
observation tower described by Julia Elwood as an "elevated gazebo" used
by patients to watch the activity on the Mississippi River and as a meeting place for the men and women in the hospital. Julia notes, "According
to some reports, it was the site of many an amorous encounter!" (*Known
Simply*, 42).

Dr. O. E. Denny
Carville, La.

Sir:—
    You, the Medical, and the Administrative Staff are cordially in-
vited to honor us with your presence at our entertainment to night.

Gabe Michael
Sec. & Treas.
W.C.C.
Carville, La.

"*Staff are cordially invited to honor us with your presence* . . ." Ordinarily staff and patients maintained a clear separation in the institute. Separate dining facilities catered to each group; laundry was done separately for staff and patients; a hedge divided the patients' living area from the homes occupied by the staff; even as late as the '70s in the Catholic chapel patients and staff sat on opposite sides and received Communion separately; and in the auditorium where movies were shown there were seats reserved for the medical staff at the back of the room. In light of the rules of segregation, this invitation from my grandfather and the "What Cheer Club" seems audacious.

Treasury Department
United States Public Health Service
Carville, Louisiana
March 2ⁿᵈ, 1925

Dr. O. E. Denny
Carville, La.

Dear Sir:—
    It is rumored that there is an opening for an appointment in the Laboratory, and I hereby tender this as my application for same.
    Thanking you in advance for any consideration given this application,

I am,
Yours truly,
Gabe Michael

"*Treasury Department.*" This is clearly a job application; thus, my grandfather uses a more formal format and style. Patients were afforded opportunity to apply for jobs within the institution: cleaning rooms in the institution, operating the elevator, delivering trays to hospitalized patients, working in the lab, and distributing medication were some of the jobs available. In the 1930s, they received pay of between $25.00 and $40.00 a month. Letters from Edmond's brother Norbert in the Louisiana Leper Home indicated that patients held jobs, but there was no mention of payment.

Dr. O. E. Denney's response follows

March 5, 1925
Mr. Gabe Michael
U.S. Marine Hospital No. 66,
Carville, Louisiana.

Sir:
    Referring to your note of recent date inquiring concerning a position in the laboratory, I have to state that arrangements for the filling of this position had been tentatively made a week before your application was received.

Respectfully,
O. E. Denney, Surgeon (R),
Medical Officer in Charge

For a period of time my grandfather was in charge of the young boys (whom he referred to as "my gang") who were patients at the hospital. The following are rules for them written in Edmond's own hand and perhaps even developed by him. They give a glimpse into the life of the young patients, some of the ways of life in the hospital, and to my grandfather's values and sense of discipline.

Rules for kids House 31
1. Rise—not later than 6:30 AM
2. Go to meals 3 times daily
3. Take Oil or medicine as ordered (Every boy to eat in one section D. Room)
4. Bathe daily
5. Keep self clean
6. Keep House and Rooms clean

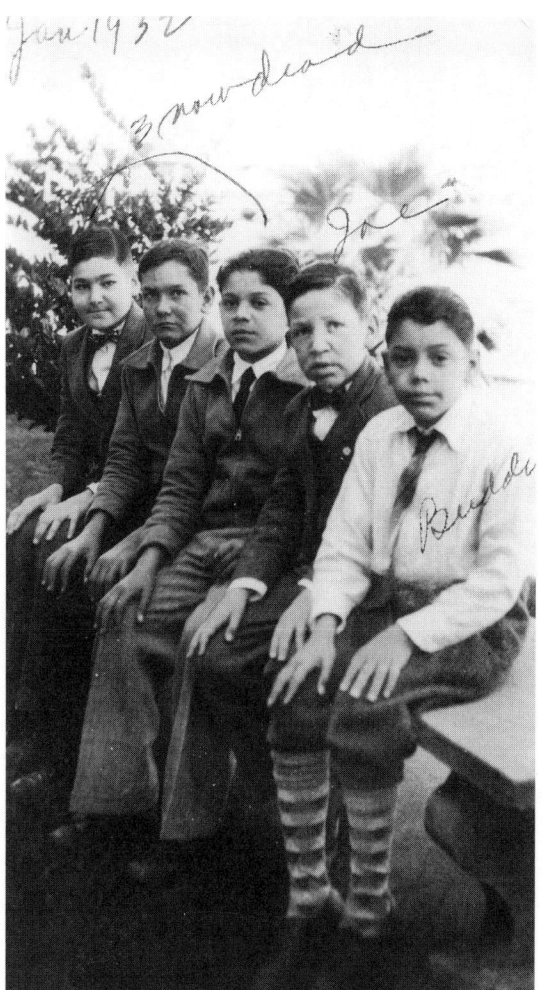

Five young men, patients in
Carville in the 1930s. (Five
Boys [patients] at the National
Leprosarium, 1932. Photog-
rapher unknown. History of
Carville, Vol. 1. Prints and
Photographs Collection,
National Hansen's Disease
Programs Museum, Carville,
LA; No. 19.)

7. No cursing

8. No vulgarity

9. No gambling or smoking

10. No loitering in Recr. Hall except hours of ____

11. Rest period after dinner to 1:30 PM

12. Respectful and polite to all

13. Not to leave house after ____PM

14. Retire, not later than ____PM

15. Attend school daily

16. Attend church services on Sunday

17. Write home at least once a month.

No exemptions from above rules without written order from a Doctor

(Signed) Gabe Michael

Carville, La.

....

Sept. 23, 1925
Dr. O. E. Denny
Carville, La.

Dear Sir:—

 Referring to my compensation claim # C-1,305,414 which has been declined on account of insufficient evidence, I enclose herewith affidavit which proves that I had symptoms before enlisting which are now recognized as Leprosy and would thank you to have my claim reopened.

Yours truly,
Edmond G. Landry

"*Edmond G. Landry.*" This is a formal letter relating to my grandfather's medical compensation so it is written and signed formally. Edmond and Dr. Denney pursued my grandfather's claim for several years but always with the same results. The Veterans Bureau found no service related connection that warranted full compensation.

LETTERS IN A TIME OF CRISIS

The letters that I have from my grandfather to his wife and family in 1928 indicate that the year was a critical one for him in Carville. Likewise, his letters to the Veterans Bureau and to Dr. Denney represent a man tortured by his isolation and struggling with his confinement. Correspondence between Edmond, the Veterans Bureau, and Dr. Denney in February and March 1928 shows both the intense darkness and the spirit of self-sacrifice that my grandfather exhibited.

U.S. Marine Hospital 66
Carville, La.
U.S. Veterans Bureau
Washington, D.C.
Feb. 22, 1928

Gentlemen:
    I would like information, or a decision, on the following questions:
    If I, as a patient in this hospital, rated total and permanent on ac-
count of leprosy, would abscond from this hospital to take treatment
at home or at some other hospital, what action would be taken by the
Bureau in regards to payment of insurance and compensation now
being paid to my wife and I under claim C 1 305 414? In other words
would payment of these be discontinued?
    In the event of death of one rated totally and permanently dis-
abled drawing full compensation does his dependent heir or heirs
continue to receive compensation? For instance, in my case, a wife
and two children. Would they continue to receive anything, and how
much?
    If possible, please mail me a copy of complete regulations.

Yours truly
Edmond G. Landry

This letter was taken seriously by the Veterans Bureau, as the following
letter to Dr. Denney shows.

United States Veterans Bureau
New Orleans, La.
March 8, 1928

Dr. O. E. Denney
Medical Officer in Charge
U.S Marine Hospital
Carville, La.
C1 305 414
Edmond G. Landry

PERSONAL AND CONFIDENTIAL

Dear Sir:

Your attention is respectfully referred to the attached copy of a letter addressed to the U.S. Veterans Bureau, Washington, D.C., under date of Feb. 22, 1928 by the above named ex-service man, a patient in your institution, and a copy of a reply addressed to the claimant this date by the undersigned.

A copy of the claimant's letter is furnished you for the reason that it is believed it is the intention of the veteran to either elope from your institution, or destroy himself.

Very truly yours,

B. C. Moore
Regional Manager

....

New Orleans, La.
March 8, 1928
[To:] Edmond G. Landry

Thru Med. Officer in Charge,
U.S. Marine Hospital, 66
Carville, La.
C 1 305 414

Dear Sir:

This is to acknowledge receipt of your letter of February 22, 1928; addressed to the U.S. Veterans Bureau, Washington, D.C., requesting information relative to your compensation status should you elope from the Marine Hospital at Carville, La., and the compensation status of your dependents in the event of death.

Your letter was referred to this office for the necessary attention and reply for the reason your entire file is contained in the regional office.

In reply please be advised that under the regulations of this Bureau, it will be necessary should a claimant who is a patient in a government hospital, leave such institution without official leave, or discharge, to discontinue his compensation, effective Date of Last Payment, for failure to cooperate; and in the event of death of a claimant who is receiving compensation on a Permanent and Total Rating, or in fact any rating, his dependent would be entitled to dependency death compensation, only in the event the claimant died from his service connected, compensable disability. If he should die from any other cause, the dependents would not be entitled to the benefits of death compensation.

Very truly yours,

B. C. Moore
Regional Manager,
New Orleans, La.

"*Thru Med. Officer in Charge.*" Although Edmond wrote directly to the Veterans Bureau their response to him was through Dr. Denney. This gives some insight into the military environment of the hospital.

Clearly, neither absconding from the institution nor taking his own life would guarantee any protection for Edmond's wife and children. Life would have to go on and it did. My grandfather may have contemplated suicide or escape but in a February letter to Dr. Denney, he was willing to be of service to the doctor and to submit himself as a human specimen at a medical meeting in New Orleans.

Feb. 20 (or 29ᵗʰ), 1928

Dr. O. E. Denny:
    To-day I learn that you desire a few volunteers to go to New Orleans to demonstrate manifestations characteristic to this disease to visiting Doctors there. I was under the impression that this convention was not until May, therefore, had not as yet offered myself to this cause.
    It is unfortunate that this disease cannot be studied satisfactorily on animals and still more unfortunate that most of the patients are so reluctant to submit to such demonstrations.

If I can be of any service at this convention or at any other time or place, I will be more than glad to volunteer. Furthermore, if granted the privilege of making this trip, and if you desire me to, after reaching New Orleans I will bring on myself, spontaneously, a lepra fever reaction, with fever about 101 to 102, active tubercles, very red; neuritic pains all over, by taking a few doses of Potassium Iodide.
At your service now or any time.

Gabe Michael.

"*Demonstrate manifestations characteristic to this disease . . .*" There are few details of the New Orleans meeting itself; however, Edmond did mention to his family that "there were those there who were afraid of us." He also indicated that he would be willing to bring on symptoms of leprosy, something he noted was possible in his 1928 letter to his wife, page 112. José Ramirez, an HD patient nearly forty years after my grandfather, described his own experience as an object of demonstration. He indicated that the occurrence was thoroughly humiliating. (Ramirez, 63)

I am not sure how long my grandfather was in charge of the Boys House. However, in October 1929 the job was discontinued and Edmond was offered other employment. My grandfather was clearly frustrated with the decision and, I believe, with the implication that he was remiss in his duties. The tone of the letter attests to his frustration.

U.S. M. Hospital #66
Carville, La.
October 15, 1929

Dear Dr. Denny:
On Saturday, Oct. 5, 1929, you decided to discontinue the Boys House which I had been in charge for the reason that none of the boys room was in order for inspection that morning, which reason was given me by Sister Martha. At this point, I wish to state that the reason the house was found in such condition is because I had told the boys that we were all to move to house 41 that morning as I had heard Sister Martha state so to Skipper on the day before. On Sunday Oct. 6th, Sister Martha advised me that my job as "Disciplinarian" had

been discontinued but I could keep on dispensing the medicines in the Mess Hall at $25.00 per month, which I refused for the reason that besides dispensing of the medicines three times daily there is plenty figuring to be done in adding up each individual patient's 3 daily doses at the end of each week. When entering each weekly amount of drops taken during said week on a monthly report sheet on which the total amount of drops taken during month is figured up and divided by 15 to be converted to C.C.s which is entered to each individual chart sheet. And besides the Chaulmoogra Oil there are seven other treatments that I have been dispensing and keeping record on. In fact, Sr. Laura who has done this work before will tell you that this job alone is worth $40.00 per month.

On Tuesday, Oct. 8ᵗʰ, Sr. Martha instructed me to explain the work to Frank Smith who would succeed me at $25.00 per month, which I did. On the next day she offered me $40.00 per month if I would continue above and in addition check up Oil Shots and keep records of same which [I] accepted. Yesterday without giving me any reasons, she tells me that Mr. Lawton would take over my job to-day and when I asked for what reason I was fired she hesitatingly replied because "We can't pay you $40.00 for that work."

I cannot understand how she can hire any one on one day at $40.00 and 5 days later fire him for the reason that "We can't pay you $40.00." I tried to see you yesterday but was told that you were busy at your office and I would not disturb you. I do not think that I was fair[ly treated] and am making this complaint to you asking you to intercede in my behalf.

Yours truly
Gabe Michael

[A copy of Edmond's letter in his file indicates that this letter had been answered in person.]

"Dispensing the medicines . . ." At least as my grandfather, a bookkeeper by training, described the job, dispensing the medicine was tedious and required a great deal of record keeping. A letter to his family in November acknowledges that he again was dispensing the oil.

"*Sister Martha and Sister Laura.*" The actions of these two women suggest that, while the Daughters of Charity were not in charge of the hospital, they had influence and a substantial amount of interaction with the patients.

Carville, La.
July 31, 1930
Prof. W. H. Hoffman, M.D.
Laboratorio Finlay
Habana, Cuba

Dear Sir:
    I enclose herewith $1.00 for which I would thank you to mail me
1 reprint copy of "Choroiditis in latent leprosy" or as many as this
amount will cover. If you have any other reprints of interest on lep-
rosy, I would thank you to mail with above instead of additional cop-
ies. If any additional charges send package C.O.D.

Thanking you in advance, I am
Sincerely yours,
(Signed) E. G. Landry

"*Choroiditis.*" Choroiditis is an inflammation of the eye, specifically the uvea. Blindness was a threat to leprosy patients and a particular fear for my grandfather so it is understandable that this article would interest him. My grandfather uses his own name and gives no indication of his position at the hospital, again for me indicating an agency of his own.

On August 9, 1930, Dr. Denney received the following letter from Dr. Hoffman:

Habana, Cuba
4 July 30 (sic)
Cerro 593 Laboratorio Finlay

Dear Doctor Denney
    I received this letter with one Dollar enclosed from Carville. I
shall always be glad to send reprints to members of your medical staff

but if the sender is not a Doctor, as it seems to me, I should be obliged if you will kindly have his letter mailed back to his address.

With my best thanks and compliments I remain
Yours very sincerely
Prof. W. H. Hoffman M.D.

Dr. Denney relayed the doctor's reply to Gabe Michael in a formal note and indicated to Dr. Hoffman that the money had been returned to Mr. Landry, a patient in the hospital. Dr. Denney's letter to my grandfather reads thus:

Mr. Gabe Michael
U.S. Marine Hospital
Carville, Louisiana

Dear Sir:
   Doctor W. H. Hoffman, of Havana, returns to me your letter of July 31, 1930, with the one dollar bill, with the request that you be informed that his reprints are not for sale and are only distributed to members of the medical profession.
   I am, therefore, returning herewith, your letter and the one dollar bill.

Respectfully,
O. E. Denney, Surgeon ®

This final undated letter to Dr. Denney from Gabe Michael presents another one of the issues that patients faced, requesting home visits, once those were allowed.

U.S. Marine Hospital #66
Carville, La.

Dear Dr. Denny:

I have written to the Board of Health for permission to make a visit to my home in New Iberia and am asking your consent to leave here on Sunday, Oct. 12, if I get approval of the Board.

In this connection I wish to state that my brother [Albert] will be in New Orleans on the 12ᵗʰ and as Eddie Darre's brother will visit him here next Sunday, I would like to know if I could go to New Orleans with Mr. Darre to meet my brother so as to save him this extra trip.

I am asking to go on a visit now, as I realize that there will be too many patients asking for leave around the Christmas Holidays.

Very truly yours,
Gabe Michael

"*I have written . . .*" By the late 1920s and early 30s patients (at least those from Louisiana and Texas) were granted limited leaves from the hospital provided they received permission from the MOC and the Board of Health for their particular parish or county.

"*Save him this extra trip.*" My grandfather had been frugal in school and in the service. Here he is concerned about saving his brother money and time by meeting him in New Orleans. David Breaux suggested that perhaps Albert was manifesting signs of leprosy and would not have wanted to be seen at the hospital.

My mother recalls that when her father visited he was accompanied by military officers, a memory that was corroborated in Betty Martin's book *Miracle at Carville*. However, there is no mention of guards in this request. Perhaps the law had changed.

"*I am asking to go on a visit now . . .*" My grandfather is clearly familiar with the protocol and the habits of the patients, and he is also solicitous of the needs of other patients. October 26 was my grandfather's birthday so perhaps he also looked forward to being home near his birthday.

A Final Letter: *Hope All of You Are Well—Love to All*

This undated letter is not my grandfather's last although it may have been during the last year and a half of his life, for the kidney condition he mentions is the one that caused his death. It is not his last, but it is for me his finest and a fitting end for his entire collection. It presents a quiet acceptance of his fate. He is a man away from those he loves but for the moment at least at home where he is.

Friday Night

Dear Folks:-

Just a few lines to let you all know that I am feeling alright. Have been going out for a walk every day this week. This afternoon I walked to my house [his cottage] in the back. On my way back I stopped at 41 house—my place—39 house Eddie M. to listen to radio & at Val's room as he had missed me at hospital. I don't feel tired. My legs are stronger and don't swell much. I just get a little pressure feeling in the chest. Besides I have earache on one side & toothache on the other. It is getting cold to-nite. Hope it clears up tomorrow.

I have not yet found out about my last kidney test. There has been so many seriously sick that I don't always get to see the doctors.

Hope all of you are well

Love to all
As ever Edmond

Friday Night

Dear Folks:—

Just a few lines to let you all know that I am feeling all right. Have been going out for a walk every day this week. This afternoon I walked to my house in the back. On my way back I stopped at 41 house - my place - 39 house Eldie M. to listen to radio, & at Val's room as he had missed me at hospital. I dont feel tired. My legs are stronger & dont swell much. I just get a little pressure feeling in the chest. Besides I have earaches on one side & tooth ache on the other.

This letter is one of my grandfather's later letters. At least for a moment he seemed at peace with his life. (Landry Letters from Carville; used with permission.)

-2-

It is getting cold to nite
Hope it clears up to morrow
I have not yet found out
about my last kidney test.
There has been to many
seriously sick that I don't
always get to see the doctors
Hope all of you are well
Love to all
                as ever
                Edmond

CHAPTER 6

Out of the Shadow: Finding Edmond

"If you ask me whom I would want to meet in heaven, I will tell you. It's Edmond Landry."
Paul Landry, Edmond's sixth grandson

I cannot know what life in our family would have been like had we not been touched by leprosy and its secrets. My mother herself acknowledges that her reticence and "stand-offishness" was in part due to the secrets she had carried most of her life. Perhaps all of us in the family would have been more generous with hugs, kisses, and physical affection had this unspoken taboo not hung over us. I have often thought that our stoicism and reserve about expressing our emotions was caused in some part by our secrets and the underlying fear that my grandmother had about leprosy. Had questions about our grandfather not been subtly forbidden, we may have asked questions about other members of our family and discovered family stories that are now lost. My brother says that the story of our family was that we did not tell stories; there is truth in that.

I also do not know how my own life would have been different had my grandfather lived unscathed by leprosy and the secrecy surrounding his existence. My grandfather died in December 1932, thirteen years before I was born. Although I searched for him during much of my childhood, it was not until I was in my fifties that I discovered him. By then I was ten years older than he had been at his death. I was no longer a lost child scavenging for her absent grandfather. I do not know what he would have been like as a father or grandfather. He had had less than five years to even cradle his own children, and although he desperately wanted a relationship with them, he was connected to them only remotely.

I like to think that he would have been a grandfather who doted on his seven grandsons and me, his only granddaughter. It is pleasant to think that we would have walked along the family property, flown kites, and ridden horses in the pasture. Had he lived in New Iberia and not died in Carville, we may have gone with him and my grandmother into his parents' home, a wood and *bousillage* structure alleged to have had massive wooden furniture and chandeliers hanging from the ceiling. The family home may not have been abandoned and we would not have viewed it with the fear leprosy had engendered in us. It would have been Grandpa's home that we could visit and explore.

He certainly would have told us stories of growing up on Spanish Lake, visiting relatives in Lafayette, and living in boarding houses while he attended school in New Orleans in 1909. Grandpa may have made a great mystery of the stranger who stole his school mate's gun out of his trunk one day in New Orleans. He may have told stories about seeing President Taft there and later Teddy Roosevelt in New Iberia. He would have taught us to strip the cane in the fields and chew its long stalks. We would have picked pecans and peaches on the family property, caught crawfish that crawled out of their holes in the spring, or explored the attic at the home on Weeks Street. Aunts and uncles from Lafayette may have visited more frequently and with less secrecy. We may have even walked with him to Estorge Drug Company where he worked and sipped fountain Cokes as we sat on chairs at the counter, our legs swinging.

But that is fantasy. My grandfather's letters show a man of discipline and drive, demanding of himself and often impatient with the system that unjustly confined him. He seems to have been a stern man who took his obligations seriously. Those same characteristics would have been with him as a parent and a grandparent. My mother, his own daughter, who was five when he left for Carville and who saw him briefly only twice more, described him as a man who "saw what he had to do and did it." That certainly describes her, too and impacted Edmond's eight grandchildren and may have indeed been an apt description of him. I do not know how he would have been as a grandfather; that I will never know. However, while I never had him as a grandfather, I do believe that his years in Carville tempered him into the person whom I admire today.

CHAPTER 7

Lives Remembered and Restored

"The only thing it is a lonesome place."
Norbert to Edmond, August 8, 1919

M y grandfather's life was always the object of my search. He was the
one I wanted to know, but I knew little of him and even less of his
siblings. In fact, I had little sense that Norbert and Amelie even existed until the family letters were found in 1977. They, like Edmond, had died before any of my generation was born, and they had been swallowed up in the
secrecy that surrounded us. I remember meeting Marie and Albert once or
twice when I was a child. Once Marie died in 1962, Albert visited our family more often. He became a participant in our family: always present for
graduations, weddings, and funerals until his own death. But silence still
inhibited our conversation and euphemism cloaked the truth. We talked
about Uncle Albert visiting from Baton Rouge, not Carville.

Because my personal interest was always in finding my grandfather,
I devoted less time to studying Norbert, Marie, Albert, and Amelie.
However, they, too, had stories and their lives deserve the acknowledgment that can be gleaned from information about them. While Norbert is
known only through his letters, we have stories about Marie, Albert, and
Amelie from their friends in Carville who were still alive when I began
my work. These friends had memories and stories about my relatives that
added to my knowledge of them. This chapter will use the existing material on Norbert, Amelie, Marie, and Albert to restore their stories that have
been silenced for too long.

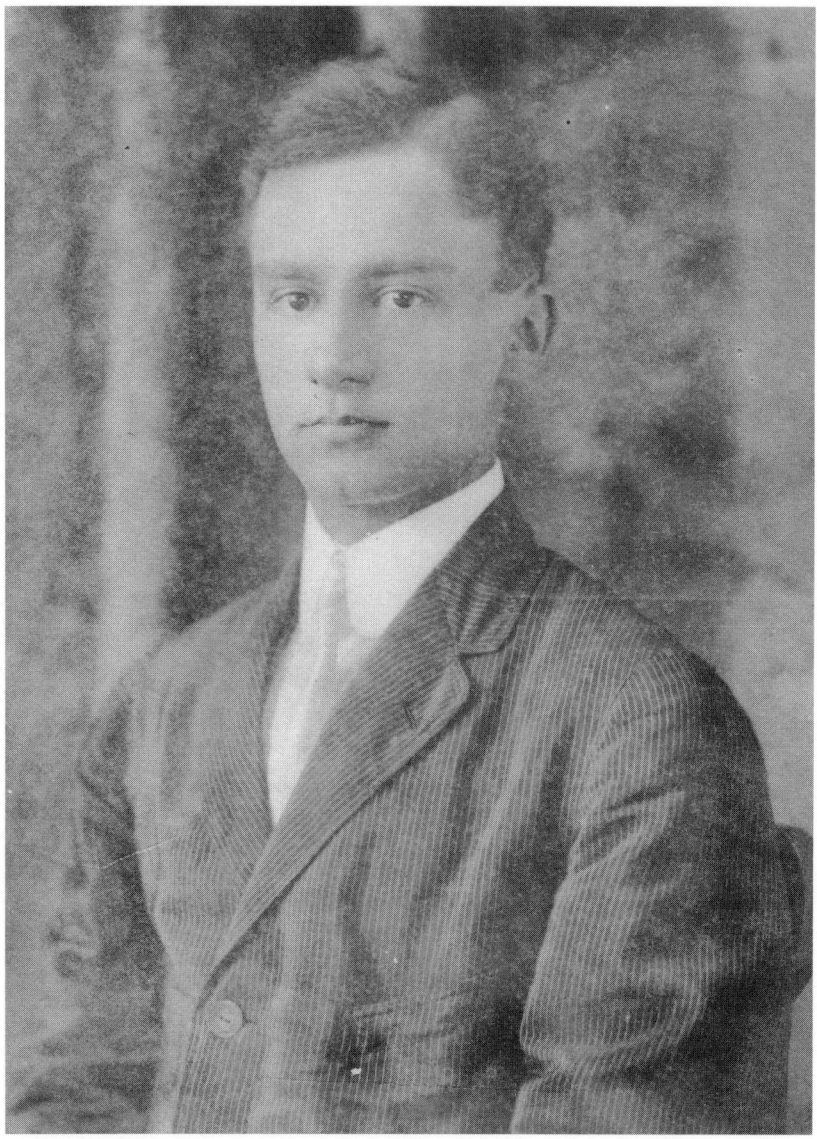

Norbert, in the years before leprosy caught up with him. In Carville, he wrote that he had a derby hat, had grown a moustache, and looked like Charlie Chaplin. (Date unknown; family collection; used with permission.)

Letters from Carville: Norbert Landry to his Brother Edmond

"With love to you one and all. I am your Brother JJ."
To Edmond, Sept. 15, 1919

Norbert Landry served in the army in France from October 1918 until his return to the States in April 1919. During that time he contracted meningitis and also showed symptoms of leprosy, a condition he may have had previously but that was exacerbated by the tensions of war. He returned home in April with the intention of working and marrying his fiancée, Louise. By July 30, 1919, he was a resident of the Louisiana Leper Home in Carville, Louisiana, the precursor of the United States Public Health Services Hospital. He remained at Carville from July 30, 1919, until his death in February 1924, eight months before his older brother Edmond was incarcerated there.

We have a total of fifty-one letters from Norbert between August 1919 and December 1924; most of them are before 1921 when the Louisiana Home came under the governance of the federal government, but his correspondence indicates that he also wrote letters to his relatives in Lafayette and for a few months to Louise. Of the fifty-one letters to family, thirteen of them were written to his brother Edmond, always with the intention that they would be shared by the family.

In his correspondence, Norbert maintains a naïve faith and optimism that prayer and medicine would effect a cure and that he would be released from the Home. His letters project his loneliness but also his trust in God, hygiene, and medicine to cure him; attitudes that are remarkably different from those of Edmond. His letters, more than Edmond's, give an insight into the day-to-day life in Carville, especially when it was the Louisiana Leper Home. Although most of the letters are to his parents, his first one is written to Edmond who may already have feared that he too would be stricken with leprosy. Certainly Edmond's isolation at home in 1923 and 1924 gave him ample time to recall and contemplate the letters from his brother.

In my room after breakfast Aug. 8, 1919
Mr. Ed. Landry
New Iberia, La.

Dear Brother;
*   I was to write before but I didn't have any stamps. So I got the*
Sisters to get me some.
*   Well I am getting along alright but the only thing it is a lonesome*
place. I take my medicine regular and my bath too.
*   I have made up friends with one of the fellows here. We go to*
church every day most. They have the benediction and the Rosary ev-
ery evening. So we have nothing else to do so we go and pray to God
for our cure. That is our only joyous pass time to go there and pray.
*   Louise sent me a novena of the St. Teresa which I say every day.*
Tell Claire I do not forget hers neither.
*   Ed. you know I should be writing home instead of you but as*
you had asked me to let you know when I would be ready for the
Typewriter, etc. I thought I would write to you instead. Show them
my letter at home and they would get of my news the same way. At
the same time I am saving a stamp. So when I write to one it will
count for all.
*   Ed. whenever you get ready to send that stuff down you can do so.*
Listen the best way is to send it Parcel Post if it don't cost too much.
This way you address it James Jackson Carville, La. but if you send
it by freight or express, address James Jackson, St. Gabriel, La.
*   I received a letter from Aunt Edmonia yesterday and a card from*
Aunt Adrienne day before. Certainly glad to hear from them. Aunt
Ed. tells me that Amelie was sick but is better now. And Papa also
had fever to 103 but was better too. Hope it was not much.
*   Well Ed. How is your little family? Hope they are all O.K. Kiss*
them all for me. And do not forget the folks at home too. Hoping to
hear from you soon. Best regards to you and all. I remain your loving
Brother, N. T. Landry

"They have the benediction and the rosary . . ." Norbert, more than
Edmond, mentions the consolation he received from his faith. Their

personalities were different and their confinement in Carville was at a different time. When Norbert first entered the Home, the Daughters of Charity were the sole administrators of the Home and had more involvement in the day-to-day needs of the patients, including their spiritual well-being.

James Jackson was the alias chosen by Norbert when he arrived in Carville. In a letter to his mother he notes that they "call us any old thing," but James Jackson was his official alias. He was also lovingly known as Cisero (and later Cisco) by the Daughters of Charity and some of the patients. He was more secretive about his condition and his residence than Edmond was. He requested that his alias James Jackson be used in correspondence and he suggested that his family come through New Orleans when they visited him so that no one would know his whereabouts. For a time he even signed his letters using the initials of his alias.

His obituary simply mentioned that he died in a veterans' hospital but gave neither the cause of his death nor the location of the hospital. His family honored his request for secrecy, but New Iberia and Lafayette were both small towns and it seems that despite his efforts people must have known of his condition.

Wednesday morning
August 26, 1919
Mr. E.G. Landry New Iberia, La

Dear Brother;
Your letter reached me yesterday noon with two others, one from Aunt Ed and one from Louise. They were very much appreciated.

I understand why mamma didn't answer my letter yet. I would have written anyhow last week but I was kept pretty busy in the kitchen.

I would have answered those letters yesterday evening but the Sister gives us little jobs everyday to clean up or cut grass or fix chairs. So she had me cleaning up under one of the houses and cutting grass around it with a few other boys.

I am getting along pretty good in shorthand. It seems to be much easier than the Spenserian [sic].

Just came back from breakfast. Had to stop writing to go.

I understand that you all are getting lots of rain, but we are not. We get a little shower once in a while but not enough to wet the ground.

Got a card from Aunt Ed. Monday and also a little box. On the card she says I am sending you a box of Shinola Polish and when I opened it, what do you think it was? Some gum. I was surely stung. Well Ed I have other letters to write so will conclude for this time. My health is O.K. and hope you are all the same. Best wishes and kisses to you one and all. From NTL.

PS You ought to see our little Chapel how beautiful it is since it was repainted. Everything shines in there. It looks like a Cathedral inside.

"Sister gives us little jobs everyday . . ." Norbert mentions on more than one occasion that he and the other patients helped around the Home. The Louisiana Leper Home administered by the Daughters of Charity was underfunded by the state, so the patients were probably not paid for their services as patients were once the Home was under federal auspices. One can argue about the injustice of this patient labor, but from the tone of Norbert's letters it seems that he entered willingly and enthusiastically into the work for the Home. If nothing else it was probably a relief from the monotony of life in Carville.

Monday morning
Sept. 15, 1919

Dear Brother;

I am just back from communion and thought I would have time to answer your letter, before breakfast. I have been taking communion every morning lately. Have finished a Novena to St. Teresa since last week. Expect to make another, which Sister asked me to do.

Ed. I have those papers to fill in. Would send them back but the Dr. will not be here before next Friday. So do not wait for same before Sat. or Sun.

Well I have my Typewriter since the early part of last week. Nothing was broken except the little ball on the right which you turn

*the roller with but that don't hurt anything. Would write with it to
you but you did not send me any paper for it. And also the book that
goes with it.*

*Well Ed. how did the storm treat you all? Hope it was not much.
It didn't blow so very strong here. We must have gotten the tail end
of it.*

Did you succeed in moving in your new house yet? Hope you did.

*How is the little family? And how is every body at home? Give
them all love.*

I am feeling pretty good these days.

I will close for this time and hope to hear from you real soon.

With love to you one and all. I am your Brother.

J. J.
xx

"*Have finished a Novena to St. Teresa . . .*" Again, Norbert's letter indicates that he was appreciative of the spiritual support offered by the Sisters,
although many of the patients of other faiths were not always as grateful
and were sometimes resentful. When the federal government took over the
hospital in 1921, the religious women became federal employees, subject to
the United States Public Health system's governance separating church and
state. They did not have the same charge of the hospital, but they did continue to offer comfort and solace in the spirit of their founder St. Vincent
DePaul. My mother to this day continues to be grateful to the Daughters of
Charity for their work and attention to patients including our five relatives.

"*Dr. will not be here before next Friday.*" During the tenure of the
Daughters of Charity at Carville, Dr. Hopkins came from New Orleans
once a week to visit and care for the patients. Norbert's letters suggest that
his visits were weekly but not always scheduled for the same day of the
week. Once the federal government took over the operations of the hospital, there were doctors in residence, but Dr. Hopkins continued his visits to
Carville until his death.

"*JJ xx*" Norbert used the initials of his alias in correspondence from
September 1919 until January 1920 when he again used his given name or
initials. In one letter he explained that the "xx" represented the initials of
his given name. Edmond never used his alias to sign letters to his family.

Sunday Evening
Oct. 5, 1919

Dear Brother;

I am sure that you are saying to yourself, "What is the matter with Norbert he didn't send those papers back"? And doesn't even write to say what is the matter. Well I thought I would write to you all when the Notary fixed the papers and sent them at the same time, which is the very thing that I will do. Will enclose them with my letter. It took a good while to get the Notary. Had to get one from St. Gabriel.

Received Mamma's letter saying that she had sent me a package but didn't get it yet, don't know why. I hope that it is not lost. Mamma asked me to let them know which way was it best for them to come see me when they do come? Well I tell you the truth I couldn't tell her exactly but I asked the Priest and he says that he thinks the best way is to come from N.O. unless they take the T.P. [Texas and Pacific Railroad] in Crowley and change at another branch before getting here. They can find out from the Ticket Agent some where. Myself I think that it would be best to go to New Orleans first as the people that know you all won't know where you are going.

Ed. this is the third letter I write with my typewriter and want to beg pardon to you for not writing the first one to you as it was my duty to do so in order to thank you for your kindness of giving me the machine. I would have written to Mama or Marie this time so as to answer their letter but as I wanted to thank you I thought I would write to you this time, and do so.

Say Ed. I want to tell you how surprised I was to see how good and well composed letter Marie writes. You know I was away for a year and had never seen one of her letter yet. But I must say I want you to give her much congratulations for me. The letter she sent me was a very nice one. I really think it beats me writing one. She tells me that she has two more years at school before finishing. Well I hope that she will do it.

There is one of the patients that ran away last Thursday night, and there is a new one that came in Sat. from New Orleans.

Say Ed. I am getting short of money as I pay to have my clothes wash and some time buy a few things for us to cook together in our kitchen. Would you send me about ten dollar bill if you please. I also had a little table fixed to put my Typewriter on which I had to pay. Or you could send me a blank check from the Lafayette Bank so that I can sign it and send it back to you to have it cashed. I have a couple of hundred in that Bank. Please send me money the quickest way. Now do not think that I want to run away. No I believe too much in God to do that. I expect to go out the right way from here.

I got a letter from Aunt Pauline and also two cans of sugar cane yesterday. The two cans were cut open and the cane was all sour and full of red spots, so I had to throw them away. Aunt tells me that Stella and Renaled have moved in their house last week.

Mamma tells me that you have moved in your house also and that she helped you all to move. I am glad to see that you are in your own home. How do you like the new place? Hope fine. I would certainly like to see it. Mamma says she likes the place very well.

Well I am running short of news so I will have to conclude my letter here.

I am feeling first rate and hope you all the same. Sending you lots of love and kisses to all of you. And hoping to hear from you soon, I am

Your Brother
J.J.

"People that know you all won't know where . . ." In Carville, Norbert was much more secretive about his condition than was Edmond who in his letters home admitted that people knew of his condition. Norbert did take steps to insure that his condition was not revealed, but his efforts were not without reason. There was at least one woman who visited the Landrys frequently inquiring about Norbert either from sincere interest or curiosity. My mother who knew the woman suspected the latter.

"There is one of the patients that ran away . . ." Norbert, more often than Edmond, mentioned specific cases of absconding. Physical conditions were much harsher in the Louisiana Leper Home—food was scarce and

treatment was limited, so perhaps there were more defections. However, Edmond might have been more reticent about this or wrote of it to Claire.

"Now do not think that I want to run away." Although Norbert witnessed many defections, his faith in a cure kept him in Carville. Sadly for him, there was no cure or release.

Wednesday 2 P.M.
October 8, 1919

Dear Brother;

I am just in receipt of your letter of the 5ᵗʰ in which you say that you didn't get those papers yet. Well you must have them by now and will see that the reason I didn't send them before is because I couldn't get a Notary quick enough.

I am sorry that I have waited that long before writing, I will try not to let it happen again as I ought to know that it must worry you all not to get any news of me. But do not worry I am feeling O.K. and am still going to communion every day.

Certainly am glad to hear that you had two raises lately. This will help you more in life. Also glad to see that you are working at the Court House every day but that surely must give you lots of work to do and keep you busy all day.

Ed. I wanted to tell you on my last letter of the 5ᵗʰ to tell mamma that I don't think that I will need my overcoat. That if she sends me my Sweater, think it will be enough. Also tell her that I didn't get the package she sent me yet. Ask her how she sent it. If she sent by freight or express, she should address it to St. Gabriel, and if by parcel post, to Carville, La. Will you tell her also to send me my two khaki handkerchiefs.

I want to thank you for those stamps which you sent me. I was not out of them yet, had one book left which one another sent me. I just got a writing tablet today from Aunt Adrienne and she also sent me some stamps with some envelopes also. I am very thankful to all those that sends me such as it will keep me from missing any.

Beings that I didn't get that package which Mamma sent me, you must say, "Well where does he get the Typewriting paper? Well

Louise sent me them a few days ago. Very nice of her too. I appreciate that very much.

I also got a letter from Aunt Ed. yesterday and one from Aunt Pauline Sunday. Was glad to get news from them. Aunt Ed. tells me that they had bad luck with the fair last Sunday. It rained all the time nearly.

Say how about some Pecans? Are they ripe yet? Couldn't you all send me some, I surely could eat some right now.

Well Ed. I think this will be all for today. Will write longer next time.

Give my best wishes and lots of love and kisses to all.

Hoping to hear from you soon, I am, as ever.

J. J.

"*I just got a writing tablet . . .*" The state run facility had no way of supplying incidental items that the patients needed since the Daughters of Charity received meager state funds and only limited support from the charity of others. I feel that this dearth of basic items may have been part of my grandfather's incentive for starting the canteen when he arrived in Carville.

"*Say how about some Pecans?*" Both my uncle and grandfather appreciated pecans from home. One letter to his family proved that Norbert was both gallant and innovative with this treasure. He gave some pecans to the sisters and sent some to the women's side of the home, but charged the male patients for theirs.

Friday Morning
Nov. 21, 1919

Dear Brother;

As we are waiting for the Dr. and I am doing nothing I thought it would be a good time for me to answer your letter which was highly appreciated.

I have gotten that package of Apples and Corn-beef O.K. and appreciate to have same except that corn-beef, don't you think that I had enough of that in the Army. Of course I gave it away to certain fellow who likes it and kept the Apples which I was longing to have some to eat sometime. I must not forget to thank you for them. They are certainly big and juicy.

Have not yet received the package which Mamma sent me a few days ago. It might do like the other one, take over a week to get here. Forgot to tell you that I have gotten a big package of cane from Laf. last week. So I want to say that I did and thank you ever so much for it.

I am doing fine with my typewriter. So far as for the Shorthand I am getting along slowly. No I do not need any typewriting paper yet.

Wrote a letter to Mamma day before yesterday but forgot to ask her to send me a pair of winter everyday pants. A kind of good one for me to go to church so that I won't have to wear my suit pants all the time. Also a pair of sleeve holders and some Ties. I have but one tie which I can wear for winter. And the sleeve holders which I have are broken.

The Priest was asking me when my Father was coming the other day? He says for me to tell him to bring him a goose when he comes over, he feels like eating some geese he said. I told him that father could send it to him by mail. So please tell papa about same. And if he does send it by mail to send it on the Priest's name Rev. A. V. Keenan not on the sister's name.

There is supposed to be a new patient coming today. He is coming on the same train as the doctor I suppose.

How is the little family? How do you all like the new home, still fine I guess. Now do not forget to send me that little kiddie's picture I am anxious to see her.

Well I am short of news so will send my best wishes and lots of love to you one and all, As ever your Brother.

J. J.

P.S. Ed. I wish you would send me a medium pocket knife, nice one now. I feel lost without one in my pocket. Sat. Morning. and didn't get Mamma's package
P.S. You will find enclosed a few medals which Sister Regina gave me to send home. So you all can divide.

"A medium pocket knife . . . I feel lost without one." There is a poignancy about this simple request from a young man who has lost so much.

"You will find enclosed a few medals . . ." The Daughters of Charity were in the habit of giving holy cards and medals to Norbert for his family, a practice that he appreciated.

> *Thursday night*
> *Dec, 18, 1919*
>
> *Dear Brother;*
>
> *Was to write before but thought Mamma would give you the news, so I put off till today. Would have written with my Typ. but it makes too much noise to write on it at night cause it wakes every body up. I would have written during the day but was kept busy all day today, painting chairs for the Sister.*
>
> *I was expecting mail from you all this week but all is in vain so far. Got a letter from Aunt A. this week, that's all.*
>
> *You can tell Papa that Father Keenan received his goose and is very fond of it. He may have written to Papa already but anyhow tell him.*
>
> *A terrible thing like to happen here last week. You know the last fellow that came in, was so disgusted and worried over his family that he took some Poison tablets. He said he was better off dead than to worry this way. But he didn't succeed. He took too many of them (they were bichlorided [sic] Tablets), made him throw up right away so didn't take effect much on him. He is alright now. He says he won't do it no more. All he ate this week was milk and the white of an egg. But he says he is mighty hungry. Good thing he says, it is the Dr's day tomorrow. [He can] change his food and eat more. I am the one that carries his food to his room every meal.*
>
> *We took another little walk through the woods last Sun. We like to take those walks.*
>
> *Ed. you will find enclosed a few Christmas cards which I am sending you all. Will you please give Uncle Henry and Uncle Filias' cards personally for me. These cards were given by the sister Sup[erior] today. Each patient got an envelope full of Christmas cards with ten cent stamps too. One stamp for each card.*

Sister Regina asked me to keep a few blank lines whenever I write home, for her to drop a few words in it also. So by doing so I will have to close although I have no more news to give you.

I am still feeling O.K. and hope you all the same.

Hoping to hear from you soon. Lots of love and sweet kisses to you <u>all</u>. I am as ever,

Your Brother,
J. J.

Postscript from Sr. Regina
With all my heart I wish you a Holy and Happy Christmas. May the Divine Infant bring you His choicest gift and blessings is my earnest prayer. I am proud of your darling son. He is so brave and good. Sr. Regina

"*Took some Poison tablets.*" Suicide was a real but little acknowledged problem in both the home and the hospital.

"*We took another little walk . . .*" In an earlier letter to his family, Norbert mentions that Sister took the men on a walk in the woods and brought some apples and oranges for them. Norbert was more of a raconteur than Edmond. There are few similar accounts with such detail in Edmond's letters. It seems that despite the harsher living conditions of the Louisiana facility, Norbert at least experienced it as a home. The United States Public Health Services Hospital #66 offered better food and more medical attention but also a more military-like atmosphere.

Wed. Evening
Jan. 14, 1920

Dear Brother;

I must beg pardon to you and Mamma both for not having written before. I've been putting off every day but this is long enough. I received Mamma's yesterday and your second one day before yesterday. Both of your letters was a surprise to me and joy at the same time. But nevertheless I am just as proud of Mamma's letter as your two for it was a nice and long one.

I showed your two letters to Sister Regina and she is just as proud as I am over it. She says she is praying for me too.

I have just taken my bath and am now lying in bed making a copy of my letter to write it on the Typewriter.

Ed. before I forget I want to tell you to take out of that check whatever I owe you. Now do not be afraid and take all what is coming to you. I know I owe you $60.00 without the last few bills I borrowed from you. I do not mind any how you take $25.00 to make it square. Are you continuing to pay my insurance for me? Please take it also from that check. By the way it is like a dream I can't remember if I refunded that money to Papa for last year's insurance when I was in the army. Ask him if I did or not. If not well pay him out of it too.

Another thing I have some money in the Bank of Laf. If you can get it out without my signature, I wish you would take it and put it all in the Bank [in New Iberia]. If you can't do it that way, well send me a blank check on the Bank of Laf. and let me know the balance due me and I shall make out the check for same.

I met one of the Sisters on the walk the other day. She stopped and asked me when my folks were coming? I said soon. She says they will surely find a great change in you when they come.

You will find enclose a little medal for T-Ni-Ni [Edmond's daughter, Leonide "Teenie"] which the Sister Regina gave me to send her.

Mamma was asking me if they had to let us know before hand when you all are coming. You can tell her that it is not necessary but it would be better. Also tell Papa that the Doctor's day is usually on the Friday but sometime he comes a day or two before in case there are some very sick patients. The last three weeks he had been irregular. One week on a Tuesday, the other week on the Wed. and the other on a Thursday. This week he is coming tomorrow. He usually comes on the evening train and gets here at about eight o'clock and the next day he makes his round visiting the patients. So he will be here tonight.

There is an old fellow who is in bed a good while before I come here. We are watching for him to die any minute. He is talking out of his head. He has been that way since Sunday. He was having convulsions all day Sunday. I thought sure he would have died during that night.

Mamma asked me something about L. L. [Louise L] but I won't tell her until I see her. I suppose you heard about it, too, didn't you? Well please do not spread it no where cause it will show for itself enough. It is a shame for what that girl has done me.

Tell Papa not to worry they do not mind us having little pets like dogs and cats. Some fellows have pet cats.

How are they getting along with the streets over there? Hope they are advancing with them.

It is ashame I owe an answer to the folks in Laf. and didn't write yet. Got a letter from Aunt Adrienne and a very nice one from Uncle E.

So as I am getting short of news, will close yours to answer Uncle Eraste's.

Hoping to see you all soon I will send you one and all lots of kisses with love, As ever,

Your Brother,
N. T. L.

P.S. Please send me a couple of calendars with pictures so that I can hang upon the walls of my room.

"*I am just as proud of Mamma's letter . . .*" Lucie Landry's first language was French, and although she read and spoke both French and English, she wrote all or most of her letters in French. I don't know if Norbert's excitement is in the length of the letter or the language in which it was written.

"*Ed before I forget . . . it is like a dream.*" I cannot imagine the turmoil and stress that Norbert had been under. In June 1918 he entered the army, was sent to France in October, contracted meningitis in early 1919, and may also have shown symptoms of leprosy in France. He returned to the United States in April of 1919 and was in Carville by July.

"*I met one of the Sisters . . . they will surely find a great change in you . . .*" Norbert's letters were often optimistic, filled with reports from the doctor and the Sisters that he looked better and was improving. It is difficult to know if these reports were genuine, Norbert's story to his family, or a desperate hope by all involved, but Norbert never did get the discharge he so desperately wanted. He died in February of 1924 of tuberculosis.

"*It is a shame for what that girl has done me.*" Norbert was deeply grieved over Louise's decision to break up with him. He asked his mother to throw away the pictures and letters that were at the family home in New Iberia and he got rid of all mementoes he had. Sister Regina gave him a rosary very much like the one Louise had given him so that he could dispense with the one from Louise.

It is unfair so many years later to try to understand or judge Louise's actions. She may have realized that there was little or no hope for a cure for Norbert, or she may have been pressured by her family to break the engagement lest her own younger siblings be at risk should Norbert ever leave the hospital. A distant relative who knew Louise's family told us that she had married, but I don't know when.

"Tell Papa not to worry . . ." Pets were allowed in the Louisiana institution but were forbidden under the harsher rules of the federal institution. Stanley Stein, who entered the Federal hospital in 1931, described his own efforts to have his dog sent to Carville. Learning that the animal was a pedigree Dr. Denney refused permission explaining that the climate was "death for pedigreed dogs. They all get fits and die." Stein could only speculate about what the climate would do to him. (Stein, 68).

"N. T. L." Norbert again used his own initials in correspondence.

Monday Evening,
Jan. 19, 1920

Dear Brother;

I am in receipt of your letter since Saturday and was indeed glad to get same but beg pardon for not answering before. I thought I would have written yesterday evening but as the Sister took us out for another walk was unable to do so. For we came back in time for supper and after supper was Benediction at about six thirty and after Benediction I felt so sleepy that I put it off till today. I also got Mamma's box of candies Sat. They are very good. Thank her ever so much for me.

Ed I am enclosing you a letter which you will oblige me in handing same to the owner. I certainly appreciate very much what they have done for me and will owe them this for the rest of my life. I am certainly thankful to them.

I also am enclosing you a letter which I got from the Gov. yesterday. It is the notice of my pension I know, but do I understand that this is for life time or what? You may send it back to me if you wish.

I wrote a letter to Nann this morning and will copy from her letter the part where I told her what the Dr. had said about me to write same to you.

Friday when the Dr. came in my room he went near the window and told me to come to the light so he could see us good. He again said to the Sister, "this boy is certainly improving." Then at night I was talking to Sister Regina a good while and during the conversation she told me what the Dr. had said about me to them. He said, "I am so proud of that boy, (and mentioned my name), to see how he has improved since he is here." This makes me think that I am well. But will continue to pray to God for my early cure. And will also go to communion as often as I can.

I have gotten myself a Rifle to shoot at the black birds and pass my time when I feel like taking some exercise. There are seven fellows who each have one just like mine. It looks like a little army when we all start out for a hunt. The only thing we can't go far enough to get any thing good to shoot at except Jay birds and Red birds. We all took our Rifles yesterday to go on our walk. We only saw a Rabbit but didn't get it.

You know the fellow I was telling you about on my last letter who we were watching to die any minute. Well he finally died last Friday. They have sent his body to his family in New Orleans.

When are you all coming over? Tell Papa that he will find a change in the place when he comes, cause they have built a new fence on the women's side. They painted it all white. And one house on our side they have repainted also.

How is the election going on over there? Tomorrow is the big day. Who are you voting for, you never told me? Papa told me he was for Stubbs. The Priest here is strong on Parker. He says Parker has a majority of about fourteen thousand votes in New Orleans.

Well Ed. I have run out of news and cannot say nothing else. So I will close in hoping to hear from you soon.

With lots of love and sweet kisses to you one and all, As ever,

Your Bro.
N. T. L.

"It is the notice of my pension . . ." Norbert seems surprised to learn that his pension will be for life. He fully expected to be cured and able to work and thus not need the pension.

"Friday when the Dr. came . . ." This strikes me as an invasion of privacy, but it may have been the informal relationship between the Daughters of Charity, the doctor, and the patients. Lack of privacy continued in the federal hospital. Patients waited for their medical visits in a waiting room separated only by a cord from the doctor's open office door.

"I have gotten myself a Rifle . . ." The imagery in this paragraph again shows Norbert's storytelling skills and for me reiterates that for Norbert, at least, the Louisiana Home in many ways had a more relaxed environment than the federal hospital.

"They have sent his body to his family in New Orleans." Many patients were buried in the Carville graveyard, identified only by number. The bodies of other patients were returned to their families for burial. Norbert was buried in the tomb belonging to his mother Lucie's family in Lafayette. (See Gaudet for a discussion of burial under the pecans.)

"How is the election going on over there?" Although Norbert had been a veteran of World War I, he, like all the other residents of the Carville hospital, did not have the right to vote. This right was returned to the patients on November 5, 1946, when a statewide mandate gave the patients their constitutional right. (See Gaudet, xi, and Stein, 236, for discussions on this.)

Sunday Evening
Feb. 22, 1920

Dear Brother; (Edmond)
   No doubt you are waiting from some news of me each day as much as I am waiting for yours every day, thought sure that I would get some kind of news from one of you all at least today but all was in vain. So I will not make you all wait any longer, will write you now. I know it is my duty to do so.
   Your letter reached me since last Sunday was indeed glad to hear from you. Did you all get Amelie's letter which I told her that I had received yours. Now I have a sad thing to tell you, I have not gotten that bunch of bananas yet. Don't know what became of them. They

must be all rotten by now. I have sold for about six dollars worth of pecans and have enough left over for my own. By the way the Priest took some pecans from me but the Sisters didn't.

Well Ed. Tell Papa that my old friend Toney is gone. He made his escape last night. Poor old man it is true that he misses his family but not more than I miss mine. There was a long time that he was telling me that he felt like leaving but I tried as much as I could to coax him to stay here long enough to get cured for he was doing splendid for the length of time that he was here but nothing doing he had it in his head that he wanted to go now so he did. He was surely a comical old man.

Ed. I am in receipt of a notice from the War Risk Insurance since yesterday which I am enclosing you herein so that you may see what is what. There is one phrase in there which will no doubt make you all open your eyes but that is not true, they do not know that I can be cured that is why they say so. By the way what did you do with the other notice I sent you?

Will you please tell Mamma that summer is coming again and I will need another summer suit if she will please buy me one (blue serge) to my size. I usually take a 30 x 29 pants and the coat is size 34. I also would like a cap over here, the one I had is all worn out.

Say when are you all coming? Mamma need not rush that suit cause there is time yet. You all may bring same when you come.

I am improving right along and hope it will continue that way. How is your little family and all the family at home? Hope they are all in the best of health.

Will close for this time as I have nothing else to say. Good luck to you and health be with you all the time.

Sending you one and all loads of love and sweet kisses,

As ever,
Your loving Bro.
N. T. L.
P.S. I see where there is thirty eight that died in New Iberia of the Flu. I see that Mr. Tilly died of it too, that is too bad.

"They do not know that I can be cured . . ." During the 1920s and '30s, cures in Carville were infrequent. However, Norbert, certainly in the first two years of his treatment, held out hope for release. The Sisters and the doctor seemed to encourage his hopes, either to bolster his spirits and theirs or because they saw progress in his condition. Edmond's letters do not indicate that he had the same belief in a cure.

"I see where there is thirty-eight that died . . ." The Great Flu pandemic of 1918 must have been still fresh in the minds of all citizens and so thirty-eight deaths in a small town would have been cause for concern.

Wednesday Morning.
May 26, 1920

Dear Brother:

I am just back from church and I want to send you this money order today no later. So will write you a few lines at the same time before breakfast. I could have sent it to you before but Sister didn't give it back before Monday noon. So you will please find enclose herein same.

I have just received my package of pecans yesterday. You will tell Mamma that the package I spoke to them [about] which I was waiting from Montgomery Ward just arrived yesterday too and yet only part of it. I suppose the other parts will follow soon.

The Doctor has changed [his] day to come visit us again, he comes at first on the Friday. They took the test from a woman on the other side last Friday. Hope my turn comes soon.

It is my turn in the dining room this week. Mr. Johnson and myself are on the same week.

Please tell Mamma that I had forgotten to tell her on my last letter what Mr. Johnson had told me to tell her. He says to tell her that he thanks her very much for what she is doing for him and he hope she will be heard in her prayers. He says if it would not be for his three little children he left behind he wouldn't worry. His Father came to see him last Monday. His visit was so short that I didn't get to see him as I was working in the dining room

Well time is short before breakfast, so will close for this time.

I am feeling very well and hope that this letter finds you all the same.

With love and many sweet kisses to you one and all.

As ever, N. T .L.

....

Tuesday morning,
Jan. 18, 1921

Dear Brother;

I received Mamma's letter a couple of days ago and was indeed very glad to hear from you all but I am writing to you instead because I want to send you my check for this Month which I just got a few days ago. I am enclosing same in this letter.

I am just back from Mass which I prayed for all the sick at home. Got a letter from Aunt A. also a couple of days ago in which she told me that the Dr. made Agnes stop school for awhile, she also said that it was unnecessary for her to ask me to pray for poor little Agnes which she is right for I say a prayer every day for her health again. I offered my communion for her last Sunday, and I am saying a Novena with Sister R. and some of the ladies on the other side.

Say by the way I also got my box which Mama and them sent me. It arrived yesterday noon safe and sound. Some of the popcorn had spilled all over the box. There was a hole in the box and a little mouse got in and ate a piece of bread off. The bread is very good not so hard. Tell Mama that I surely do like that Calendar. Thank her very much for me. That face on that is so pretty. I mean beautiful. It favors some one I know very much, you know who I mean don't you?

Mamma asked me how the roads were over here and well you can tell her that they are pretty bad right now but if the weather keeps up this way they will be good again soon. We haven't had rain for nearly a week. They will have to hire an Auto, cause the Sisters do not send the Truck any more.

Well I have no more to say for this time will close. Hoping to hear from you real soon.

With oceans of love and sweet kisses to you one and all. Kiss Ti-Ni-Ni for me will you. Wish I could see her now.

Your loving Brother
N. T. L

"That face on that is so pretty." This passage leads me to believe that Norbert never stopped loving Louise.

Thursday Morning
Mar. 10, 1921

Dear Brother;
    Your letter of the 7th was received since a couple of days ago and was highly appreciated by me. Yes you are right I understand very well why you couldn't come to see me and also knew it from Mamma and them. I am sure you have lots to do now as your Boss is away.
    No doubt you have realized and thought what day it was today. The 10th of March, my Birthday. What do you think of that. It seems as if it was yesterday that I was Fifteen years old and look what I am today, 26.
    Dr. Denny is back from Washington since last night, with lots of good news to our interest. He came around this morning to see my old men and mentioned that he had gotten much more than he had asked for over in Washington in line of money and different things for the interest of the place. He says that the Red Cross is going to send us fourteen Phonographs, one Player Piano and two Standard size Motion Picture Machines. I tell you that this little Dr. is putting this place up to date, and that is a great thing for us. We are surely thankful for that. But I myself I hope that I don't have to stay here much longer.
    I suppose you have read in the papers about that fellow Willard Cantiliver who had run away from here about one year ago to stir up the Gov. in Washington for a pension. Well they held him up there all that time and now that the Gov. has taken this place over, they sent him back here again. He arrived here Monday night at about seven thirty with another fellow by the name of Charles Young who

had been in Washington for a few Months also. The Dr. is wait-
ing for twelve or fourteen more patients from Boston today or tomor-
row. He is rushing to build some Temporary Houses to receive many
more, soon. They are hauling some portable houses since a couple of
weeks, which he will use for these Temporary houses.

Please give this letter to Mamma and them so that I will not have
to write them an extra one this week. This one I know can bring them
all the news that I can gather around here.

Sister Regina gave me a very nice picture to hang in my room, for
my Birthday today. It has a very pretty frame to it.

By the way Ed. I wish you would send me a couple or more (so I
won't have to bother you as often) bars of shaving soap, also a box of
cigars please for me for Easter. I am plum out of shaving soap, and
by me asking for those cigars you all might think that I am a great
smoker but don't you think so. Just once in a while, like that.

I thank you ever so much for that Typewriter piece. The one that I
have pinned is still holding so I will let it stand until it breaks again.

Well as I cannot find any more to say, will close for this time. I am
very well and hope that this letter reaches you all and finds you all in
the best of health.

With love and sweet kisses to you one and all, as ever

YOUR BROTHER, N. T. L.

P.S. I didn't think it was any use to ask if Amelie was well cause I
got a letter from Aunt A. also the same day with yours in which she
tells me that Papa and the family were over there last Sunday. That
means she is well now.

Thursday night, seven o'clock

I have received Marie's letter at noon and very glad to hear from
her like that every week. Tell her I will answer it the next time I
write. Also tell her that I understood what she meant right away when
she said that the Banks would be closed four Months day for day
from the inauguration day. Yes the Banks are all closed every day on

the Fourth of July. That was a pretty good catch just the same. I don't know what made me think of the fourth of July so quick.

I also received my scarf pin and those good cakes which I am most sure that Claire had sent me. Thank her or who ever sent them, ever so much for me. I appreciated that very much. I don't mean to say that Claire sent the pin too, no I know cause Marie tells me that it was them. I love the pin too. It is very beautiful. Thank them for it also. I have looked at the paper that was wrapping the box of cakes over again and saw that it was from Claire. I was so anxious to open it up that I didn't look who it was from. Thank her a million times more for me.

Well I have no hopes of getting that chicken which Mamma sent me, cause I haven't received it yet.

I wish that You all would put the price of the things you send me so that if some body asks what it cost me I know how much to say. I wanted to sell the collars Mamma sent me the other day which were too large for me and I didn't know the price.

"I understand very well why you couldn't come to see me . . ." This is the only clue Edmond ever visited Norbert in the hospital. I am inclined to think that if Edmond did visit his brother at all, the visits would have stopped when Edmond was first diagnosed in 1922.

"I suppose you have read in the papers about that fellow Willard Cantilever . . ." Willard Cantilever was one of the early activists for the Carville patients. John Early was another one.

"Dr. Denny is back from Washington . . ." Dr. Denney was the (MOC) Medical Officer in Charge of the United States Public Health Hospital which began its governance of the Louisiana Leper Home in February 1921. Under the auspices of the state of Louisiana, the Home had been badly underfunded, but with the advent of federal operations Carville began to see an influx of more patients from throughout the country and more monies for the hospital's operations. In a letter to his family Norbert remarked about the quantities of food that the patients ate after the federal takeover: eggs every day, milk three times a day, potatoes, and even fish and ice cream. He was so excited by the latter two items one evening that he forgot to take his medicine.

Although Norbert remained hopeful to the end of his life, he died of tuberculosis—not leprosy—in February 1924, only eight months before his brother Edmond entered the hospital.

The Final Three Siblings

Amelie (aka Emma Lee Michael), Marie, and Albert were the last of the Landry siblings to enter Carville. Amelie died in 1940, five years before I was born, but I knew Marie and Albert. Sadly, the family taboo about leprosy kept me or any one in my generation from knowing their stories.

Because there are far fewer family letters from Amelie and Marie and none from Albert in Carville,[1] we do not have the same opportunity to discover their stories as written in their own hands, but we do have snippets from the letters that exist and memories from people who knew them. In those stories about Amelie, Marie, and Albert some themes are evident: involvement in the Carville community, humor, faith, and generosity, patterns that were also evident in the letters from Norbert and Edmond.

AMELIE LANDRY

> *"I will have to see the brain Dr. when he comes."*
> Amelie to family, December 1934

Amelie was the youngest in the Landry family and in 1934 was the first of the last three siblings to go to Carville. My generation knows less about Amelie than any of the other siblings. She died before any of us were born and had stayed at the family home most of the time, coming into town only rarely. Even my mother knew little about her, and was not aware that Amelie was in Carville until after her death there in 1940. In her father, Terville's, 1936 obituary, Amelie is listed as a survivor living in New Iberia although she had been in Carville since 1934.

If our family's stories were the only information about her, Amelie would have been a mystery, but her friends in Carville and remnants of her few letters afford us a picture of her as a self-effacing, lively young

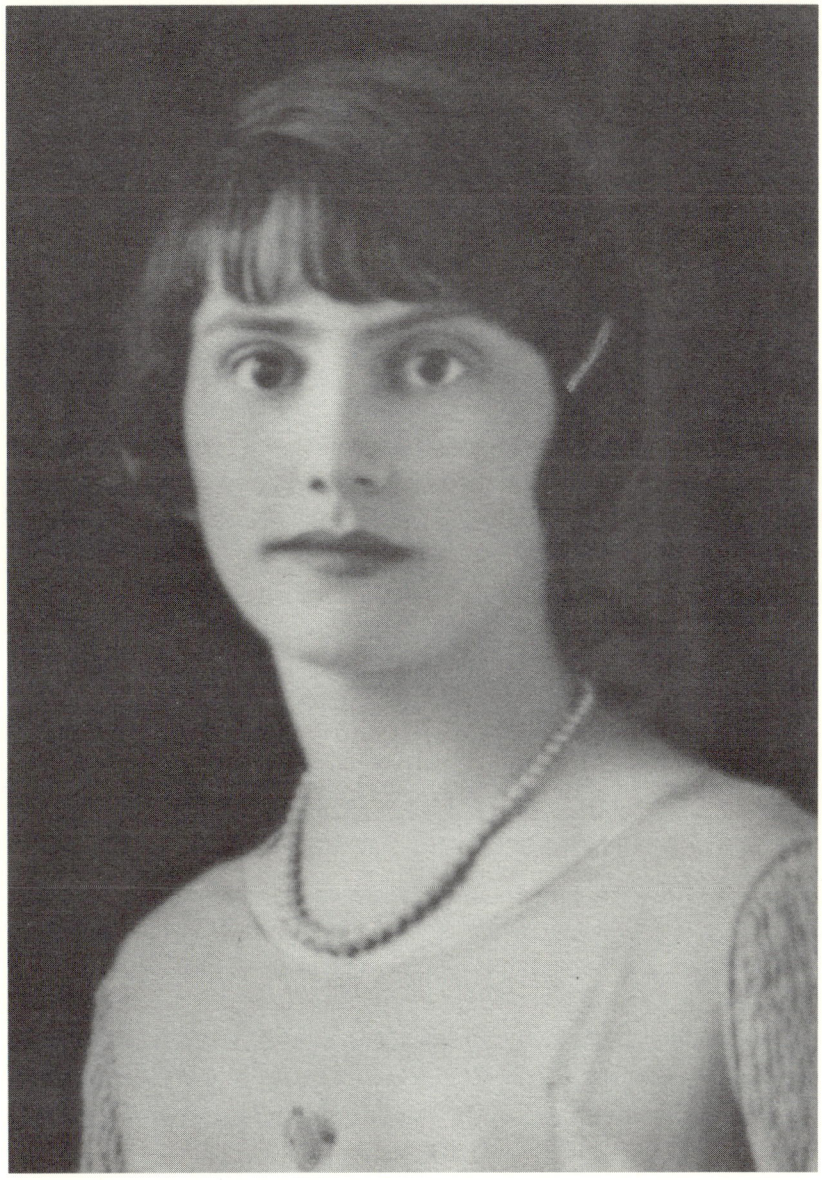

Amelie Landry was a beautiful young woman whose face, but not her spirit, was scarred by leprosy. (Date unknown; family collection; used with permission.)

woman, involved in the Carville community, strengthened by her faith, and strongly committed to her family.

In a letter to her family in December 1934, only three months after she arrived in Carville, Amelie proves that she can laugh at herself and enjoy providing laughter to others.

> *My brains were not at work properly. . . . Well the whole . . . is that I went in the wrong house last Fri., and it was in a men's house, imagine my embarrassment. I was coming back from the hospital Fri. morn. and I entered 28 house which is the men's house just before ours, went to room four, pushed on the door it wouldn't open, I pushed and pushed again finally I decided to call Bobbie (the orderly), and when I did, some man came out of room 8 and asked who I wanted, when I looked up and saw him, I then realized I was in the wrong house. Oh! boy did I get a laugh, and everybody else. I came home and told the story. I had the whole house in an uproar. They all tease[d] me and say I will have to see the brain Dr. when he comes. Well anyway it made us have something to laugh about. I guess I had the [Christmas] program too much in mind.*

When Amelie entered Carville in September 1934 she already had fifteen years of knowledge of the place, a familiarity bred of the long stays of both Norbert and Edmond. Consequently, she talks easily in her letters about fellow patients such as Felix and Skipper, men who had been Carville friends of the family for many years. Elsewhere she acknowledges changes that were happening to Carville, noting that "you won't recognize it around here."

Anecdotes from Louise Ann, a patient with Amelie in Carville, portray her as personable and popular, and perhaps spoiled, not surprising for the youngest child in her family. Louise Ann said that both Amelie and Marie played the piano beautifully, but Amelie was the friendlier of the two. Louise Ann also told me before her death that she had learned to fry chicken from Amelie. As Louise Ann tells the story, Amelie said she felt like eating fried chicken. When Louise Ann asked who was going to fix it, Amelie replied, "You are. I'll show you how."[2] Louise Ann cooked the chicken according to Amelie's directions and at her suggestion even added garlic to the hot grease for flavoring.

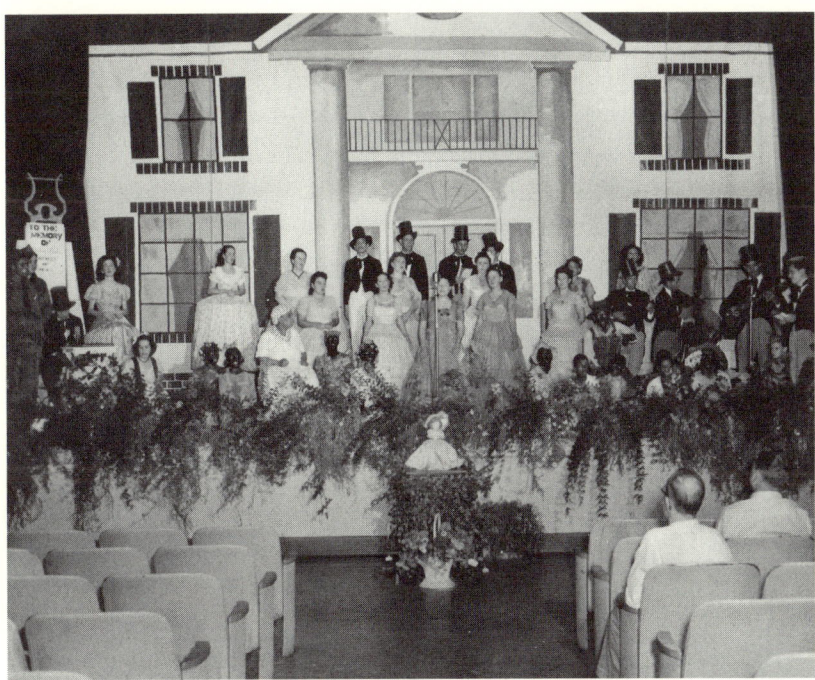

This elaborate pageant presents an interesting cultural portrait of the Carville community, which was an ethnic blend of men, women, and children from, among other places, the United States, Puerto Rico, Japan, and China. Here the performers—all patients, white, black, and black face—are involved in a presentation of the Old South. (Date unknown; family collection; used with permission.)

Amelie was engaged in the activities and work of the Carville community, participating in the Christmas pageants[3] and perhaps taking piano lessons from Sister Laura. Although I do not know what work Amelie did in Carville, after her father's death she sent home money she had made to have Masses said for him. Later, again according to Louise Ann, Amelie worked and saved her money for a death mask for her burial; this is no doubt because of the severity of her disfigurement. The one picture from Amelie's medical records shows much more severe symptoms of leprosy than did pictures of her other siblings. The one picture looks as though she had been severely burned and shows her unrecognizable except for her eyes. Mary Ruth came to Carville in 1939 and recalls caring for Amelie in the hospital when she was already badly disfigured. She had been a beautiful but sickly child and had manifested symptoms of leprosy as early as

1923, three years before she graduated from high school. Yet she did not become a patient in Carville for another eleven years.[4]

Certainly a major trial for Amelie was the sudden loss of her father in April 1936, two years after she had entered Carville. Terville Landry died only days after swallowing a fish bone which lacerated either his esophagus or intestines.[5] Amelie did not attend the funeral, but her letter home to her family after his death resounds with grief and faith.

Dear Mamma:—

Oh! God has taken papa away from us, it is hard I know but we just have to accept God's will and make the best of it. I know you all didn't want me to know, but I just couldn't go any longer the suspense was driving me crazy, I just had to know and I was prepared for the worst after reading Marie's second letter. But Mamma don't worry about me. I'll be brave and take it like a soldier, so don't worry. They all took good care of me last night. Maggie slept in the room with me, I had a fairly good night. Sr. Zoe said she would have a mass said as soon as she could and I am enclosing ten dollars that I made last month for you to have masses said too.

Marie, Albert and Sadie [Albert's wife], oh please take good care of mamma for me don't let her worry over me too much.

Oh Uncle Henry [Terville's brother] you will help console the family. I know it is hard for you too, but with our faith in God we can bare anything.

May God bless all of us in our sorrows and may he take his soul straight to heaven.

Tante Adrienne [Lucie's sister], I know too I needn't ask, you all will take good care of them all for me and help mamma have courage to bare such a shock.

Prend courage mamma, le bon Dieu nous la laissez avec nous longtemp. Que Jesus crucifé have mercy sur son ame.

With deepest sorrows I remain Your sorryful child

Amelie

The final letter in Amelie's collection gives an insight into the politics of the Carville community and also addresses an issue that Edmond had also indirectly addressed, the possibility of a cure on the outside.

Aug. 9, 1939

Dear folks:—
Well we had the visit of a big shot to-day, an inspector from Wash.
I guess he came to investigate into last week's troubles[6] and more
maybe. I haven't heard what the outcome was. . . .
    It goes to show you, you can stay out of here and get well as well.
A woman was brought back Monday that had run away about seven
years ago and they can't find the germ on her. Isn't that fine?

Love, Amelie

MARIE LANDRY

> *"There was a single red rose left on Marie's grave every year on her birthday."*
> Marie's niece "Teenie," in conversation with the author

Amelie suffered the disfiguring ravages of leprosy, but like Norbert, she died of tuberculosis on September 24, 1940, eleven months before Albert and Marie, the last of the Landry siblings, were hospitalized there. Norbert, Edmond, and Amelie had each been alone during their stay in Carville. Marie and Albert, the ones to live in Carville the longest, entered the hospital at the same time. I was acquainted with both of them since they visited my grandmother. "Carville" had been a euphemism for the hospital where my relatives died and also the unmentionable disease that they had. Ironically, however, when we talked about Marie and Albert we used an additional euphemism: we said they were visiting from Baton Rouge.

Although I had met Marie on one occasion, my knowledge of her comes from her letters and anecdotes about her from friends in Carville and my mother. Marie was the middle child and oldest daughter in the Landry family. She was nearest in age to Albert whom she considered her special gift since he was born two years after her on her birthday. She was the

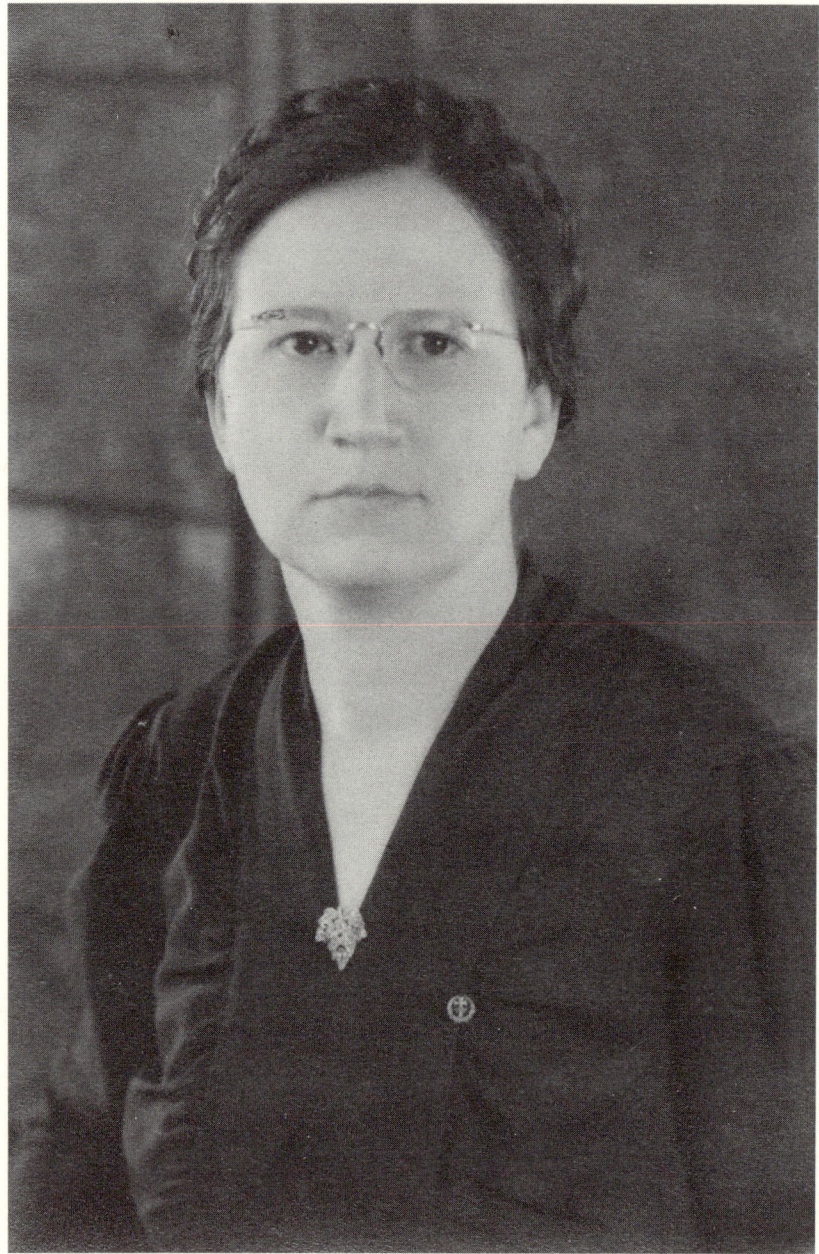

Marie Landry, prior to her diagnosis with leprosy. She was the businesswoman in the family, working outside of the home and attending to her mother's finances even after she went to Carville. (Date unknown; family collection; used with permission.)

correspondent in the family, writing frequently to Norbert, Edmond, and Amelie after they left home. Marie was also the businesswoman who cared for her mother's correspondence before she went to Carville and for the disposition of the family property once she and Albert were hospitalized. She lived at home, caring for her mother after Albert moved away, Amelie left for Carville, and their father died. I presume that either Marie or her mother had saved the family letters from Norbert, Edmond, and Amelie, and Marie brought them with her to Carville.

She, unlike Amelie, held a job outside of the home, working for the telephone company in New Iberia. She had access to a car and was generous in offering transportation to the Sisters of Mt. Carmel who lived in New Iberia and taught at the Catholic girls' school, Mt. Carmel Academy. It was her regular presence in town that led to her being reported to the medical authorities in Iberia parish. She was required to report to the hospital in Carville after it was reported by citizens in New Iberia that "Marie B. Landry has a case of leprosy, and that she is constantly in contact with people on the street and in the stores" (Dr. C. D. Mengis, Iberia Parish Health Officer, to Superintendent, U.S.P.H. Service Leprosarium, June 10, 1941, Marie B. Landry medical records).

She and Albert[7] went to Carville by August but not without some delay. When authorities went to the family home in August of 1941, expecting to find Marie and Albert ready to report to the hospital, they found the house empty and locked. Marie and Albert had disappeared. They had apparently gone to Texas to settle their mother, Lucie, there. Lucie's widowed brother and unmarried sisters lived in Lafayette and the families had been close, but the fear of leprosy was too great. There may have been room in their hearts for Lucie, but not for the contagion she might have carried. Lucie lived for a time in Texas cared for by a woman from Lafayette. When the woman moved back to Lafayette, she moved Lucie with her and cared for her until Lucie's death in February 1944. Neither Albert nor Marie were able to attend the funeral, but their sister-in-law, Claire, sent them a long and comforting letter about the services.

Marie and Albert were hospitalized in time to take advantage of sulfone treatments, the miracle at Carville, which occurred in the early 1940s. Consequently, they showed fewer effects of leprosy. Marie's letters from the 1940s show her to be engaged in the life of Carville while also maintaining her connection to New Iberia. An undated letter from her gives an indication of a typical day in Carville and also indicates her involvement with the rituals of her faith.

> *For instance to-day, I got up at 6 or 6:30 went to breakfast at 7 and that takes over a half hr. standing in line and getting served and then eating, from there, we went as our Custom every morning after breakfast and also supper to say our rosary at church. Then we go for contrast bath at 8:30 and that takes over half hr. and then we take the shots from Dr. Joe [Dr. Johansen, a well-loved doctor at Carville] which starts sometimes close to 9:30, before you finish and come to your room it is close to 10 o clock or more. Then comes the fixing and cleaning of room plus washing your clothes that would fade if you sent it to the laundry. Rest a little afterwards followed by dinner at 11:30 when we seldom leave dining room before 12:15, pass for the mail at canteen, then today pass at reading room to bring back a book. At 2:20 novena at church (every Tues.) to Our Lady of the Miraculous Medal, which finishes about 3:00 before you get to your room and rest awhile it is time for supper at 5 o'clock (They stress on rest) and after supper dress for the show (three times a week Tues, Thurs. and Sat) and sometimes ball game on the other days. In between time Sister Laura is giving me piano lessons and there is practice also. So this is the routine of the days, varying a little.*

She had her days in Carville well organized, but she also kept in touch with New Iberia. In March 1947, she requested that Claire send her the New Iberia paper and the New Iberia magazine published annually for the Sugar Cane Festival. In the same letter she agrees, for both herself and Albert, to arrangements that would give her nephew and niece, Booz and Teenie, the family farm.

> *We agree with you that Boozoo should not be looking elsewhere for a farm when he owns part of one already. What could we do with a farm and not have someone on it that has its interest at heart, and who should we want to own it besides Booz or Leonide.*
> *Knowing we can keep the house[8] in case we ever need it and also the oil rights helped us to make this decision.*

She had connections with New Iberia that continued during her years in Carville. My mother recalls that one of Marie's friends from New Iberia used to visit her in Carville, and every year on Marie's birthday someone placed a red rose on her grave.

While in Carville, a male patient showed interest in Marie, but she evidently did not return his attention. Mary Ruth recalled that the young women in the house in which Marie lived would spend time giddily spying on the men in their house that was directly across from the women's. Marie, who may have been older than the others (she was thirty-eight when she entered Carville) and definitely more reserved, did not seem to share their curiosity.

Little else is known of Marie's life in Carville. Ray, also a Carville patient, remembered that at one time she operated the hospital elevator, and I believe that she had also worked for the *Star*. Family pictures show her participating in the services in the Catholic Church and in the elaborate pageants staged and directed by Sister Laura. Hansen's disease was treatable by the time Marie and Albert entered the hospital, and it was not leprosy that killed her. Sadly, by the time that she and Albert could have received a release from Carville, Marie was almost completely blind and suffering from a "chronic brain syndrome of unknown origin" that made it impossible for her to care for herself outside of the hospital. By the end of her life, Marie, who had been a competent and intelligent woman, was in her own shell, walking around like she did not know what was going on. Julia, a friend and younger patient in Carville, remembers that she would walk with Marie to the chapel for daily Mass. One day Marie was giggling and walking slower than usual. When Julia looked down, Marie's underpants were wrapped around her ankles. Julia had Marie step out of them and stuffed the garment into her purse. She and Marie finished their walk, still giggling. Marie died in 1962. Like Norbert, Edmond, and Amelie, she died far too young but was remembered by her friends and loved by her brother Albert.

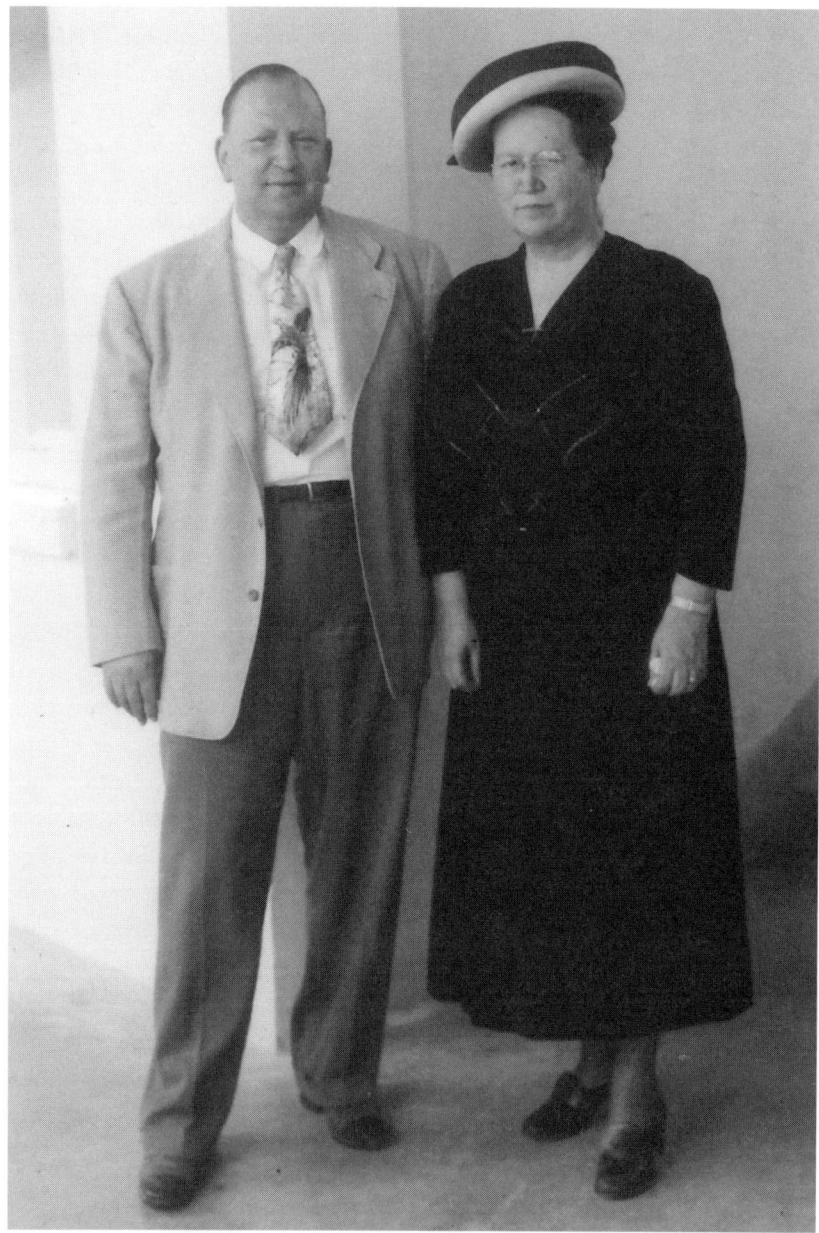

Marie and Albert entered Carville just before the new sulfone treatments for leprosy were proving successful (some said "miraculous"). There were more opportunities for patients to leave the hospital for outside visits. Marie and Albert traveled to visit relatives in Texas and Louisiana. (Date unknown; family collection; used with permission.)

ALBERT LANDRY

"Albert was a man with an easy style."
Albert's great nephew, Michael, to author

Albert's Carville friends told us that they believe that Albert would periodically quit taking medication for Hansen's disease to insure that he would test positive for it and be unable to leave the hospital and thus be available to care for Marie. This was the clearest but hardly the only evidence of Albert's generosity, which was perhaps his greatest characteristic. When I have asked former patients about their Carville memories of Albert, all of them acknowledged his generosity. In a recent email, Julia told me,

> He was a very quiet and gentle man and very generous. The patients knew that he had money, so many of them went to him for loans. I don't know of anyone who wasn't helped by your uncle. And I'm sure that not all of the borrowers paid back the loans.

My brother, Michael, confirmed that image: "At Uncle Albert's wake patients approached Mamma and me to express their appreciation for his generosity." Other patients who had been released from Carville recalled that when they would return for treatment, Albert would often give them rides to Baton Rouge if they needed them. One remembers my uncle taking him to buy fireworks that he needed for a stand he owned. A couple who met in Carville, and who were much younger than Albert, noted that he was something of a father to them. In a 2011 email, the wife told me,

> He was a kind and generous man. He treated me like his own child. . . . He was good to me and my husband and also to my children when he would come by our house. The start we got in life he gave us. Till today we still miss him. I named one of my sons (I have three) after him.

In a phone call, her husband reiterated Albert's generosity, noting that Albert had made it possible for them to buy their first house. He also taught the man to play golf and gave him his golf clubs when the couple left Carville.

José Ramirez met Albert when he entered Carville as a young man in the late 1960s. He recalls now that

> Albert would quietly donate generously to the Mexican Club when someone desperately needed funds to travel home for a funeral or some other emergency, to the Lions Club when someone was also in need, and to other causes that helped patients who had little or no financial resource. . . .

In the same reminiscence to me, José noted that when he decided to marry Magdalena (the young woman he had left back in Texas) he was the beneficiary of Albert's largesse. As José remembers,

> I shared with Darryl, Albert, Milton (the "three amigos"[9]), and Mary [my friend Mary Ruth and Darryl's wife] that I was going to propose to Magdalena before I even told my parents. They were elated because they came to see her as a daughter. Magdalena loved spending time with them and listening to their stories, some so unique that it was difficult to separate fact from fiction. Once the proposal, marriage plans, and relocation to Baton Rouge were finalized, I realized that I had no way of bringing Magdalena from Arlington and hauling all of her belongings. Without hesitation the three amigos organized a trip to Arlington, TX, rented a hitch, and Albert said he would cover all of the expenses. The four of us traveled to Texas, picked up Magdalena and her belongings and dropped her off at the apartment I had rented for her to live in until we were married. The three amigos were very protective of Magdalena and threatened to kill me if I did not return to my assigned room at the hospital every night until after we were married. They also made arrangements with Freddie, the front gate guard, to monitor my departures and returns.

I, too, can attest to my uncle's generosity. He attended the high school graduations for me, my brothers, and cousins, gifted us with his quiet presence, and gave us generous gifts at that time. At his death all eight of us were each left a generous sum of money. When my father was hospitalized for a prolonged period, Uncle Albert offered to help with our family's financial expenses. He was also generous to the Sacred Heart Catholic chapel at the hospital. He donated money in honor of the Landry family for a stained glass window. The window is in honor of Our Lady and respects the long connection that the family, especially Albert's mother, Lucie, had to the Blessed Mother.

As generous as my uncle was with his money, he was also frugal—tight, actually. He played bourré and poker regularly with other patients. He would play in the games that were for small change, not the ones for high stakes. People who told me about his generosity also remembered that when he would lose he would sulk. Again, we, his great niece and nephews, were beneficiaries of this for at his death we each received some of "Uncle Albert's change."

Albert was generous with his money and with his friendships. He maintained contact with high school classmates and established friendships with other patients in Carville. When Albert entered Carville, he became a resident of a community he did not choose. He and others of his generation were forced into the institution,[10] yet they made lives for themselves and friendships with their compatriots. Mary Ruth and Daryl were among Albert's closest friends throughout his life in the hospital. There were others, but this couple I knew and loved. José also attests to the friendship that they and Milton, another patient had. José's reminiscences tell of a group of people who shared love and humor with one another and whose love spilled over to touch him as well. His emails gave me a new picture of Albert and insight into the community in Carville.

I first met Albert approximately six months after I arrived at Carville and was assigned a room in House #23. Darryl and Mary Broussard agreed to my parents' request to serve as surrogate parents as they had done for many other young patients. Before his death, Darryl started using his real name of Wasey Daigle from Lafayette. They invited me to their cottage in the back for supper and I quickly accepted. Carville was a very busy place during the week but a ghost town in the evenings and on weekends. Those of us who ate at the "patient's dining hall" would disappear into the sanctuary of our rooms or rec hall after the early 4:30–5:30 meal. Therefore, having a home cooked meal at 6:30 pm was a real treat.

I walked slowly to the Broussard Cottage [Darryl and Mary Ruth's Carville home[11]], across the road from the then abandoned cottage where Stanley Stein lived (he died one month before I was admitted). I did not have a bicycle and it was too difficult to maneuver the hand-propelled wheelchair down the gravel road, so I walked gingerly to the cottage.

As I walked in, the Broussard's Chihuahua attacked me and actually bit my leg. Albert snapped at the dog and she quickly ran to his side. The dog would do the same thing every time I went to visit the Broussards. Darryl introduced Albert as the "richest but cheapest son of a gun at Carville," and Milton as "the laziest man in all of Louisiana." They both described Darryl as the "biggest liar in the world," and the "luckiest for finding a blind woman to fall in love with him." Mary was not blind, and none of the adjectives used to describe the "three amigos" was true. They enjoyed teasing each other tremendously and would have supper together every evening. The only time they were not eating Mary's cooking was when Albert "went across the river to visit family" or when Milton was sick (he would not visit his family in San Antonio).[12]

Living in the cottages meant having access to rations but Albert and Milton would always pitch in with some groceries. Darryl hated chicken from the time he was in the infirmary for months on a "chicken diet" and Albert and Milton loved chicken. Darryl claimed that he was "experimented on by some fools who thought eating chicken would kill the bacilli." Their arguing would go on for hours while Darryl smoked Kools and Milton his Winstons. Darryl would always sit at his recliner, Albert at a love seat facing the combination dining/living room with the vicious dog on his lap, and Milton sat on the couch. I would usually sit on one of the dining table chairs with Mary in a large couch chair with rest arms so high that she appeared lost.

All of them were old enough to be my parents and with many stories to tell. Albert was the most secretive but occasionally divulged information about his family. In my eyes, he was a big man[13] who loved his coats and hats, making him look even bigger than he was. He favored dress pants that seemed to be from the '40s and '50s, giving him much legroom. Darryl would allege that Albert would only wear secondhand clothes as he was too cheap to spend a nickel. Albert would simply laugh and stated that millionaires did not like to show off their wealth except in front of pretty young things. Albert would often tell Darryl that when he died he was going to have all of his money placed inside the casket because if he left any to Darryl he would foolishly spend it all on booze and women. Darryl would counter that he had only eyes for Mary and was "too beat up" to enjoy drinking any more. Each would have a comeback for everything and I learned to appreciate the genuine love they had for each other. Milton had a slow drawl and being hard of hearing he would often doze off while the other two tried to outwit each other.

Albert was hardly seen during the day as he stayed in his room in House 16 most of the time and would venture out to the Broussard's in the evening. He drove a big car, which Darryl said he bought from a junkyard. This obviously was not true as his car, either a Buick or Cadillac, always looked new. The three of them became friends at a young age and in spite of their major differences in personalities, they got along like brothers. They knew each other's secrets, faults and strengths and quietly loved and respected each other. I was never able to joke like they did without feeling that I was intruding into sacred turf.

Albert lost part of his youth when diagnosed with HD, but he found an extended family and learned to love them as much as his blood family. Mary and the three amigos are all deceased but the memories that we have of them will never die. To this day, Magdalena has a photo of her and Mary by her nightstand and we often recall the wonderful evenings we had with all of them. Magdalena still cries about the sacrifice they all made on our behalf.

When he entered Carville, Albert did indeed lose part of his youth and the life he had made for himself. He had moved to Opelousas sometime in the late 1920s, worked as a lineman for the phone company, and married Sadie before his confinement in Carville. They had no children and Sadie remained married to him until the mid-forties, when she requested a divorce, which my uncle granted, and then remarried, although I believe he never stopped loving her. His life changed but he entered into the community that became his: participating in the Lion's Club, serving as King of Mardi Gras, in later years traveling with friends, and availing himself of opportunities to help others.

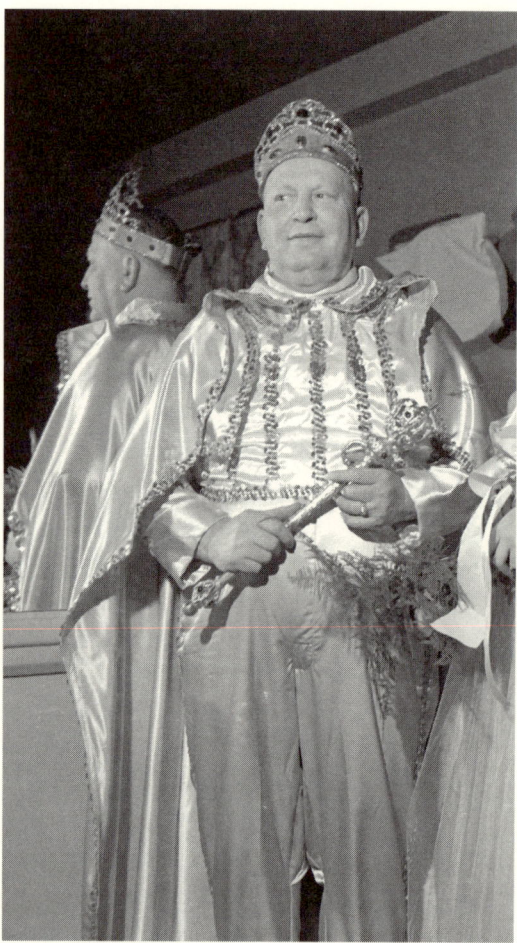

In his life Albert was a generous and noble man. Here, as King Albert, he quietly reveled in his role of monarch over the elaborate Carville Mardi Gras celebration in 1954. (King Albert, Carville Mardi Gras 1954. Johnny Harmon, photographer. Carville Mardi Gras 1954. Johnny Harmon Negative Collection. National Hansen's Disease Programs Museum, Carville, LA; JH120–96.)

My brother, Michael, recalls Albert as a man with "an easy style." He remains amazed at the lack of visible bitterness shown by Mary, Daryl, Milton, and Albert. He told me recently that when he and Sheila, his wife, were first dating, they met Albert for dinner at a Baton Rouge restaurant. Albert's first question to Michael before Sheila arrived was, "Does she know where I am?" Michael assured him that Sheila did. When they left the restaurant, Sheila kissed Uncle Albert. She had no fear of his condition and she embraced him as the person he was. That sealed for her a special affection with this man who had so much love to give. She was, in Erving Goffman's words, a "wise person" (20) who accepted Uncle Albert for who he was and he always remembered that.

As I finish this work, I trust that this story will bring Norbert, Edmond, Amelie, Marie, and Albert out of the shadow which has veiled them for too long. I hope that in listening to and telling their story I am also in some small part telling the story of others who were separated from family and community because of the quality of their skin or the secrets that surrounded them. In an email to me, José Ramirez sums it up: "Leprosy can force systems to do everything possible to make those of us affected by the disease to become invisible, but our brothers and sisters with the disease help us to resurrect the uniqueness of love and family." They need not be hidden in shadow any longer.

CHAPTER 8

Epilogue: My Journey out of the Shadow

"My family has begun to speak more openly about our grandfather Edmond."
The author

In writing this book, I intended to let my grandfather's story be told in his own words without the interruption of too much analysis or theory. However, my writing was shaped by my academic studies and that bears acknowledgment. In this chapter, I will look at my own journey and some of my research, recognizing some of the theories and analysis that informed my work and gave context to my family's narrative.

When as a child I sat cross-legged on cold linoleum in my grandmother's dark hall, I was looking for my grandfather. I fantasized that a picture of him or note by him would suddenly fall from a dusty book on the shelves I scoured. As I grew older, I wanted to find not only my grandfather but also a meaning to the silence that seemed to invade our family and kept us mute about this man whom I could only imagine. I found his mandolin and fiddle but no pictures or notes from him, and for many years the silence won. I held onto my secret search as though it were some sort of talisman that eventually weighed heavily on me. Even though I desperately wanted to know him, I was silent, on occasion paralyzed, about speaking of him when friends outside the family could have revealed him to me. My fantasies of him and the family taboo against speaking about him were stronger than my search for him. Yet that search continued slowly. To this day, I remember the moment when I first discovered my grandfather. I was sitting on an orange Naugahyde couch reading Stanley Stein's memoir *Alone No Longer* when I discovered this passage, "Gabe was probably the only altruistic character. . . . There were plenty of patients happy to do a good turn for a friend. Loyalty was, in fact curiously common. But a desire to work for the common good was not. Gabe Michael was a native Louisianan and a World War I veteran. He had been in the wholesale drug business before Hansen's bacillus caught up with him" (53). I knew instinctively that this man was my grandfather. That nugget sustained me for another twenty years.

When I finally began to tell my family story, the writings of Sissela Bok and Carl Jung helped me to understand my attachment to this secret. I learned what Bok called the "feel of secrecy." "We are all in a sense, experts on secrecy. From earliest childhood we feel its mystery and attraction. We know both the power it confers and the burden it imposes . . . But we come to understand its dangers, too: how it is used to oppress and exclude" (Bok, xv). Jung, too, helped me to recognize both the value and peril of secrets: "In small doses, the poison may be an invaluable medicament, even an essential precondition of individuation" (CW, vol. 16, par. 124). But he warns, "Nothing makes people more lonely and cut off from the fellowship of others than the possession of an anxiously hidden and jealously guarded secret" (CW, vol. 4, par. 432).

My experience of secrecy left me isolated but also strangely connected to the stories of others whose lives had been enmeshed in secrets: other Hansen's disease patients, holocaust survivors and their families, persons of color passing in a white world, Japanese detainees in World War II, adoptees searching for their biological roots. I felt an affinity with these stories, for they too were about lives unspoken. I experienced both this connection to the secrets of others and reticence about my own secrets well into my adult life. My studies helped me to realize that I had become attached to my secrets and later to my grandfather's letters as some sort of entitlement.[1] I saw these letters as a collection that was uniquely mine. In fact, the letters were not mine alone; they had a long and complicated ownership history that challenges me even today.

When the letters from my grandfather were finally uncovered in 1977, I did not read them immediately. Other life issues were distracting me, and I had become enchanted by my image of my grandfather and perhaps fearful that the man I met in the letters would not live up to my fantasy. I read the letters almost twenty years after they were discovered. When I finally sat down with the big blue binders that contained my grandfather's story in his own hand, I was captivated. I was once again the nine-year-old child finding my treasure, but I was also the woman who could now give form and meaning to my grandfather's life and to my own. I used my penchant

for scholarship and my desire to further my education to frame the life of
the man who had fascinated me for so long. There was a book in his letters
and I was going to write it. I discovered and used scholarship that explained
his situation and enhanced the meaning of his life. Theories of entitlement,
secrecy, stigma, trauma, memory, and narrative gave context to my search.
My grandfather's life, I discovered, had a universal context and meaning
that scholarship helped me to plumb.

My grandfather, like others in Carville, experienced stigma in full force.
Leprosy patients were ostracized, incarcerated, and abandoned because
of the quality of their skin and the assumption that immoral behavior had
caused their condition. They shared a "spoiled identity," the term Erving
Goffman used in the title of his book on stigma. As I discovered, it was
this stigma that contributed to the institutionalization of leprosy patients.
They were incarcerated[2] so that "normals . . . [were able] to arrange life
so as to avoid them [the stigmatized]" (12).[3] Ironically, this incarceration
did give HD patients a community of their own where "the stigmatized
individual can use his disadvantages as a basis for organizing his life, *but*
he must resign himself to *a half-world* to do so [italics mine]" (Goffman,
21). My grandfather lived in this "half-world," but also in the world seen
by Gaudet as a folk community. "They were part of a true folk community
at Carville—isolated from the rest of the world with their own traditions,
celebrations, stories, and views of the outside world" (20). Edmond's letters attest to this community and signify that he did enter it: participating
in its events and organizing service activities. But he did face the "half-life"
of the stigmatized, separating his family life from his Carville life. At the
same time, he admitted to his wife that he spent years trying not to enter the
Carville community, "the land of the living dead" (to Claire, June 1928).

My mother (as well as her mother and brother) also suffered from stigma. They were "obliged to share some of the discredit of the stigmatized
person to whom they were related" (Goffman, 30). My mother (who was
the only one alive to be interviewed[4]) recalled being whispered about as
"that little girl whose father has that bad disease." She recalled other instances of being brought to tears by a classmate who told her that her father was not in the hospital but in the crazy house, and having to explain
to another friend that her father's condition was not seriously contagious
and that it was safe for the friend to associate with her. On more than one
occasion, she told me that she and her brother Booz were close because

"we had each other." The experiences were painful and made my mother standoffish most of her life, but they also made her what Goffman calls a "wise person," one of those "sympathetic others who are ready to adopt his [the stigmatized person's] standpoint in the world and to share with him the feeling that he is human and essentially normal in spite of appearances and in spite of his own self-doubts" (19–20). My mother's experience of stigma and her knowledge of leprosy made her tolerant of others and more compassionate to their pain. She was always accepting of those with Hansen's disease, including her own aunt and uncle and their friends in Carville. She used to mention the deep pain she felt when she would see men and women with leprosy standing at the bus stops in New York City, ignored by drivers who refused to give them rides. It took me longer to acknowledge that my own secrecy about my grandfather was connected with a feeling of stigma. While I did have dear friends with HD living in Carville, my reticence about my personal story kept me essentially stigmatized.

Perhaps even before my mother experienced the stigma of leprosy, she, along with her family, had experienced trauma when her father kissed them all goodbye and left. I cannot imagine the adult pain of my grandmother and grandfather; I can fathom even less the traumatic experience of my mother who as a five-year-old was being separated from her father who was to "go to a hospital to get well." Cathy Caruth's description "that trauma is not experienced as a mere repression or defense, but as a temporal delay that carries the individual beyond the shock of the first moment" (10) is apt. My mother carried that trauma well into her later life when at eighty, at the request of her family and Marcia Gaudet, she finally spoke of her father's departure, her few memories of him, and her life after he left home. In August 2000, my mother sat with Marcia Gaudet, my nephew Christopher Manes, and me,⁵ and told her story. She was generous and responsive to Dr. Gaudet's questions, but still clearly controlled the story. As my mother later told me, "No one had ever asked me [to tell my story]," so now seventy-five years after the traumatic experience, the "delay," my mother did so. The five-year-old girl finally had her say. She, her children, and grandchildren were part of what Marcia Gaudet calls "an even larger group of people [who] are still being affected by the trauma of Carville. These are the children, grandchildren, and even great-grandchildren of people who lived through the stigma of being diagnosed with leprosy. A diagnosis of leprosy affected the entire family. The patient was taken to Carville, but the family was left to mourn the loss, almost always in silence—public silence, if not private silence" (Gaudet, 169).

This experience of trauma is what Marianne Hirsch calls "post memory" which "characterized those who grow up on a narrative that precedes their birth, whose own belated stories are evacuated by the stories of the previous generation shaped by traumatic events that can be neither understood nor recreated. I have developed the notion in relation to children of Holocaust survivors, but I believe it may usefully describe other second generation memories . . . of traumatic events" (Hirsch, *Family*, 22). I use the concept of absent memory also in Hirsch as significant in the lives of my own and succeeding generations of the Landry-Manes family. Hirsch describes the work of Nadine Fresco as "interviews with others of her generation whose parents *never spoke* [italics mine] of their abandoned world . . . and who thus have almost no access to the repressed memories that shaped them" (243).

My mother and my generation experienced the secrecy of post memory and absent memory, but our stories were not obliterated. As I discovered interviewing my mother, she had clear, well-formed kernels of narrative that had been with her all of her life. These memories included her own childhood memories and the reported speech of others.[6] As she finally told her stories, she added glosses and tag endings to explain her narrative (Bennett, 417) and to forgive and excuse those who had made her feel pain and stigma as a child. Her narratives are more than rote stories, however; they have become for her acts of intimacy and creation. They were stories she *wanted* to tell. Sandra Dolby Stahl, whose writings informed my work, suggests, "People tell stories to be listened to. . . . [W]hen people tell personal narratives, they offer listeners an invitation to intimacy" (*Literary Folkloristics*, 37).

My mother lapsed into dementia shortly after I completed my studies in 2007. Since then I have come to appreciate even more the profound gift this reticent woman gave her father, me, and her other descendants. Her stories were a gift for me, but they were creative and transformative for her. She became someone who "*was* but is now changed" (Stahl, 22). In her book, *Violence: Empowerment through Narrative*, Elaine Lawless notes: "To tell our stories is to re-create ourselves. The power of narrative comes in the act of telling our stories, breaking the silence, narrating a life, constructing a self" (160).

These narratives from my mother, the letters and life of my grandfather, and my own writing can be appreciated as what Hilde Lindemann Nelson calls "counter stories."[7] She defines "a counter story [as] a story that resists an oppressive identity and attempts to replace it with one that commands respect" (6). Nelson notes that such a counter story "positions itself against a number of master narratives: [which she describes as] the stories found lying about in our culture that serve as summaries of shared understandings" (6). Master narratives about leprosy have flourished. Patients have been treated with fear or condescension because of the prevalence of false knowledge about their condition. It is seen as a bad disease, highly contagious, and inherited. From medieval and biblical times and even earlier, those with leprosy were feared and assumed to be unclean and morally degenerate. The disease, even today, is a cultural metaphor for outcasts and the untouchables. Tasteless jokes about lost limbs still abound and even people sincerely interested in knowing about the disease reflect false information. Hollywood still uses the "L" word and demeaning stereotypes of the disease.[8]

My mother must have heard all these stories about her father's disease and in her silence may have seemed to be accepting them. However, the testimony of her life spoke otherwise: her reception of her aunt and uncle and their Carville friends into her home and life, her quiet, unspoken acceptance of her father's condition, and finally in her old age her openly told accounts of her pain when unfounded stories about leprosy had swirled about her. My mother's very act of retelling her stories was one of "narrative repair" (Nelson, 9). She claimed her position not as the little girl whose father had a "bad disease" but as a woman who could see clearly that the stories she had endured were "nothing." Once my mother began to speak about her father, she started to speak openly and with frustration about the master narratives, the medical misinformation, she had heard: "They said it was contagious but it wasn't. They said it was hereditary but it wasn't. It was nothing." On one occasion, after she had voiced these sentiments I asked her, "Mamma, how does that make you feel?" She looked at me directly with her clear, unblinking eyes and said forcefully, "Like s--t," an epithet she had never used before or since and one that she refused to let me print but one which for me spoke of a damaged identity and a narrative repair. The lies and misinformation of the master narrative, not leprosy itself, made her feel like s--t.[9] By professing her feelings and the fact that the stories she heard were "nothing," my mother claimed her own counter narrative.

This book of my grandfather's letters and life presents his counter narrative. As my grandfather's letters attest, his life in Carville was impeded by the constraints of his condition and the master narratives about it. Nelson acknowledges, "How freely we can exercise our moral agency is contingent on a number of things. . . the form of life we inhabit, the niche we occupy in our particular society; the practices and institutions within the society that set the possibilities for the courses of action that are open to us" (xi). These constraints, Nelson suggests, can cause a person to absorb the stories of others creating an "infiltrated consciousness" (xii). As I read and reflected on my grandfather's life and letters, I discovered a man who despite his circumstances fought to maintain his own identity and tell his story.[10] He refused to fall prey to the lethargy of the institution. He spent time helping those needier than he, starting a canteen and the "What Cheer Club" for the benefit of the patients, planning and participating in events that helped make the hospital a community, offering himself for medical research, independently researching his condition, and advocating for himself and the patient population. In his letters to his parents and siblings, he recounted, without self-pity, his activities in the hospital. In the two extant letters to his wife, he argued powerfully for his rights as her husband and the father of their children. He used the most up-to-date medical knowledge to present his case and to discredit the cultural myths of his time. He managed his life on his own terms, created in his letters and life his own counter narrative, and clearly lived what Arthur W. Frank would call "a good life while being ill" (Frank, 156).

In my research, it was Frank, even more than Nelson, who gave me a specific theory of narrative as it related to the sick and thus to my grandfather. Frank's 1995 work, *The Wounded Storyteller: Body, Illness and Ethics*, was written long after my grandfather's death and did not deal with Hansen's disease, but it helped me to see the ethics of my grandfather's life. "Living this good life," as Frank describes it for an ill person in remission, is not a life of ease or of obedience to medical authority but rather obedience to one's own truth. It is the challenge of living ethically and responsibly for oneself and others. Frank suggests that the role of the ill in the remission society, the person who is well but never cured (8), is not simply to survive, for that "does not include any particular responsibility other

than continuing to survive" (137). The ethical role of the wounded storyteller is one of witness and desire. For Frank, telling one's story means
witnessing to one's life, however piecemeal, chaotic, painful, or discredited
that life might be. Bearing witness is testimony to the dignity of all human-
ity. Bearing witness is one task that Frank sets for the wounded storyteller;
desire is the other. For Frank, this means "desires become responsibilities:
what is *good* to want for oneself and others" (156). My grandfather's life
was a witness and an active cry of desire for his rights and those of his fellow patients. My discovery of Frank's work gave me a model for viewing
my grandfather's life.

I completed my studies knowing that my grandfather had been spoken
about, but he had not yet spoken. I set about the task of editing his letters, thus giving him a voice, a chance to tell his story in his own words.
Ironically, as I end this work I realize that my grandfather still eludes me. I
cannot imagine the anguish he felt that October day when he left his family, never to live with them again. Edmond could say that he missed home
cooking, but I wonder what must have been the depth of his emptiness
when he sat down in a dining room to eat institutional cooking that was often in his estimation "no account."[11] He relished food from home but it was
still not a meal at home. My grandfather had been a successful businessman and family man, but in Carville he was, like others, "a poor 'leper,'"
an object of fear and scorn or of condescending compassion. He had been
a homeowner and bookkeeper in a wholesale pharmacy, but he was now
earning $25.00 a month to distribute patients' medications. He had been a
Knight of Columbus and an upstanding member of the Catholic Church in
his local parish, but in Carville he was a man who exhausted prayers and
novenas to countless saints begging for the love of his wife. He was a man
who had taken comfort in his faith but for a time abandoned it, feeling be-
reft of its consolations, unworthy of its graces, and able to trust only in the
mercy of God.

I do not know my grandfather any more than any of us can know another person but I believe his letters have brought him closer to me and out
of the shadows. My scholarship has brought me a greater appreciation of
the themes that shaped his life. Only now as I bring this book to a close can
I understand the fuller meaning of the title I chose. I originally called the
book *Out of the Shadow of Leprosy* for my grandfather and his siblings, but
my generation too has come out of the shadow. I am no longer the curious

nine-year-old sitting in a dim light searching for her grandfather, nor am I even the graduate student writing on a topic about which I was passionate. I am a woman engaged in this story—which is in some part my story as well. I can speak much more freely about my grandfather without euphemisms and explanations.

Others in my family have begun to speak more freely as well, acknowledging the confusion or pain we had in the years of silence about this man, our unknown grandfather. We admit the shock we felt knowing we were referred to in our hometown as the "'leper' Landrys." We admit now, as my brother Michael does, that ignorance, not leprosy, was the real sickness. Like my cousin Paul, we can speak proudly and publicly about our grandfather. Paul speaks because of his passion for this subject and because he does not want his own children and grandchildren ignorant of their relatives and burdened by secrecy. We have developed a website www.lepro sysecrets.com to share our story, to invite stories from others, and to mitigate the ignorance that still exists. We can laugh somewhat ironically at the story still told today that horses on the family property wore handkerchiefs over their nostrils to protect them from leprosy. This story, told to us by a veterinarian recalling the accounts he had heard, is patently false and medically ignorant. There is no human-to-animal transmission of the disease and there have been no successful lab tests to inoculate any animal, except the armadillo, with the disease.

Only recently did I become aware of just how much my own attitude and conversations have changed. I was giving a reading at a public event recognizing black authors. I chose to read an excerpt from Ernest Gaines novel *A Lesson before Dying*, the story of a young black man as he faced death for a crime he did not commit. I have long admired Gaines's work because of the dignity of his characters in the midst of the undignified treatment they endured. I see my grandfather's life in terms of dignity in demeaning circumstances, but I had never openly made the direct connection between Gaines's work and my grandfather's life. I introduced my reading by saying publicly and proudly, "I chose this reading because it speaks of a young man's courage to live and die like a man. In 1924, my grandfather, Edmond Landry, was incarcerated in the United States Public Health Services Hospital because he had leprosy; I see his story in much the same light."

Notes

1. In the early 1900s, there was pressure within the federal government to create a national institution for the treatment of leprosy. The congressional will to create an institution was there, but no state wanted to accept such a hospital in its backyard. Louisiana did not have the ideal climate for the treatment of the disease but it did have a state institution. This underfunded home, the Louisiana Leper Home, was purchased by the federal government and in 1921 became the United States Marine Hospital #66. Over the years it changed names several more time, finally becoming known as the Gillis Long Hansen's Disease Center. I refer to it as the United States Public Health Services Hospital #66

2. Leprosy and the more odious term "leper" are fraught with stigma. The words still cause pain among those who have suffered with the condition. During the period that is covered in this work, leprosy and "leper" were the operative words of the condition. My grandfather in his letters used the terms "leprosy" and "leper," although his brother Norbert apparently did not. When Edmond used the latter, the term revealed the anguish he felt. I use the words when Edmond did or when they are historically necessary, but even then I use quotations to delineate the term "leper."

3. In 1873, Armand Hansen discovered that leprosy was caused by a bacillus, Mycobacterium leprae. However, the transmission of that bacillus remains a mystery today. (In a letter to my grandmother [one of two that are extant], my grandfather questions whether the bacterium is indeed the cause of the condition.)

4. The "hole in the fence" was an actual hole in the institution's security fence that itself was topped with barbed wire. The hole allowed patients to leave the hospital out of sight of the security guards. The PBS documentary *Triumph at Carville* films the brother and sister reminiscing as they stand at the hole in the fence. The documentary also interviews their parents who were still living when the documentary was made. In her book, *Carville: Remembering Leprosy in America*, Marcia Gaudet relates stories told by patients who left the hospital through the "hole in the fence" for evening getaways and for longer escapes from the institution.

5. Betty Martin's memoir *No One Must Ever Know* chronicles the life of her and her husband, Harry, after their release from Carville in the 1940s. They were free but still living under the specter of discovery.

6. A 1947 editorial by Stanley Stein in the *Star* noted that early discharge papers were "prominently marked . . . P.H.S. 'Leper' . . . [and had] attached a clinical photograph of the discharged, the kind that would make a passport picture look glamorous" (6:5, p. 12).

7. In her preface to the text, *Feminist Messages: Coding in Women's Folk Culture*, Joan Newton Radner suggests that for women "coding—covert expressions of disturbing or subversive ideas—are a common phenomenon in the lives of women who have so often been dominated, silenced, and marginalized by men" (vii). Ours was a matriarchal family but the public narrative about leprosy at the time could have marginalized my grandmother, great-grandmother, and mother and above all made them wary of my questions that they could not or would not answer. I adopted a similar coding of my own later in life, using Carville as a euphemism for leprosy and Hansen's disease.

8. Norbert, the first of the family to enter Carville, was the only one who resided at the Louisiana Leper Home, the state-run facility that became a federal institution in 1921. Between 1919 and 1977, there were only three years when a member of the Landry family was not interred at the hospital.

9. "Carville" is a term that here refers to the institution for the treatment of Hansen's disease including the hospital, the patients rooms, all additional buildings on the grounds, and living quarters for the lay and religious staff. It is of course the town in which the hospital is set and for my family the euphemism for HD.

10. In his work, *Defacement: Public Secret and the Labor of the Negative*, Michael Taussig calls public secret that which is "generally known but cannot be spoken . . . [and is characterized by] knowing what not to know" (50).

11. This is a quotation as I remember it from poet W. S. Merwin in a PBS interview with Bill Moyers. I don't remember the occasion or date of the interview, but I have not forgotten the quote.

12. To date, this seems to be the only such collection of family letters from Carville. The letters from Edmond include letters to his parents but only two remaining letters to his wife. Norbert's letters are to his parents and to Edmond, but he indicates that he wrote other letters as well. José Ramirez had letters from his time at the hospital, but to my knowledge there are no other collections from 1919–1932.

CHAPTER 2

1. My grandfather frequently uses a colon and dash as his punctuation for letters. For me it represents an urgency and purpose in his correspondence.

2. The letters in this book, the Landry Letters from Carville, LLC, are in the possession of the Landry-Manes family, and are used by permission of the family.

3. Bahon, who was a rival during school, remained a friend to my grandfather. He became principal at the high school attended by my mother and her brother. My mother recalls that Mr. Bahon had one leg shorter than the other and walked with a cane, which he would use to "hook" students who were misbehaving in the hall. She also remembers his kindness to her, teaching her math courses that were not in the curriculum so that she would be prepared for college. When I asked her if Mr. Bahon demanded more of her brother, perhaps as a form of some kind of respect for their father's values, she responded, "Booz could get away with murder." My mother told me that when her father died in Carville, Mr. Bahon called the family and spoke to my mother, then thirteen, telling her that he had known her father. .

4. This typewriter was serviceable for many years. It was used by Edmond at school in Soulé and probably by both Norbert and Edmond in Carville.

5. Marie and Amelie did continue their piano studies, as friends who knew them years later in Carville commented on their ability to play the piano

6. When Saint Peter's College, a secondary school for boys opened in 1918, Edmond paid Albert's tuition, a gesture he kept up during Albert's entire high school education.

7. Although Louise was never identified as Norbert's fiancée in any of his letters to his family, it seems clear that she and Norbert had been intent on marrying even before he left for the service. She wrote to him while he was in the service and when he first arrived in Carville.

CHAPTER 3

1. An irony of the institution of the United States Public Health Services Hospital was that with its establishment, leprosy patients were required by federal law to enter the hospital. Prior to this, the laws were less stringent since they lacked the force of the federal government.

2. Arthur W. Frank's 1995 work does not deal specifically with leprosy but by implication says much about the fate of those incarcerated for the disease. *The Wounded Storyteller: Body, Illness, and Ethics* describes members of the "remission society" as "all those people who . . . were effectively well but could never be cured" (8). They had lost their passports in the land of the healthy and lived on "permanent visa status" (9). Frank cites cancer and multiple sclerosis as two such conditions; I see leprosy in the same light. In the 1920s, patients were rarely, if ever, cured of the disease even though it could be in remission for periods of time. When my grandfather was diagnosed with leprosy he had to, by law, enter the Carville hospital, so he was part of what I call the "incarceration remission" society.

3. Norbert died in February 1924, one month before his twenty-ninth birthday and eight months before Edmond entered the hospital. Norbert was buried in the Landry family tomb in Lafayette, Louisiana. Edmond probably did not attend the funeral, but my mother, barely five at the time, told her grandson Christopher Manes that she remembers being lifted up by her French speaking great Aunt Adrienne to view Norbert in his casket and told, "*Regardez.*"

4. In the 1940s, it was the report by an anonymous citizen in New Iberia that necessitated the examination and incarceration of his sister Marie.

5. From Norbert's letters, it is clear that family visited him, but it is not as clear if Edmond was among those visitors. He was married with children and a wife who feared leprosy and by 1922 he himself had the disease. It is plausible that he never visited his brother in Carville. If, however, he did visit, those trips must have been a painful foreboding of his own imprisonment.

6. Until 1921, the Daughters of Charity had been the primary caretakers of the home. Once the home became a United States public health hospital, these religious women became federal employees.

CHAPTER 4

1. Betty Martin, in her book *Miracle at Carville*, written years after her incarceration for leprosy, relates her first night in Carville caught "in the grip of nightmare." Particularly upsetting

for her was seeing a patient she had only just met, "her distorted face was before me and her voice was in my ears. 'Look at me. Look at me'" (10).

2. During the early years in Carville, patients were encouraged to choose an alias so as not to bring discomfort or embarrassment to their families. Norbert had been known in Carville as James Jackson and Edmond was Gabe Michael; their sister, Amelie, took the name Emma Lee Michael. Despite my grandfather's alias, my grandmother always addressed her letters to him as Edmond Landry. It is not as clear that he used his real name in the return address on his letters home, although this is my mother's memory.

The policy of changing one's name has been fraught with lost identities even today. Stanley Stein, a noted activist in Carville, received international attention and awards, but never under his given name, Sidney Levyson. My friend Mary Ruth and her husband used aliases for much of their lives in Carville. When travel restrictions for patients were relaxed, they realized they lived under aliases in Carville but traveled with documentation giving their real names. At that point, late in life they assumed their real identities. "Betty Parker" was the alias of a beautiful young debutante who entered Carville in the 1920s and later married Harry Martin, also a Carville patient. They lived their entire lives inside and outside of Carville using their aliases Betty and Harry Martin. Writing under her alias, Betty chronicled the couple's lives in her two books, *Miracle at Carville* and *No One Must Ever Know*. The books were well received and did much to enlighten the public about Hansen's disease, but at her death Betty Martin, the author, was nowhere acknowledged; her obituary gave only her birth identity. Now, however, if one Googles "Betty Martin" it is acknowledged that this was the name of Edwina Parra, a New Orleans debutante who was sent to Carville.

3. See Gaudet's *Carville: Remembering Leprosy in America*, "The World Downside Up," for an account of Mardi Gras in Carville.

4. Newspaper articles of the time eloquently described the beauty and grace of the institution, ignoring the fact that such rhetoric was no comfort to those imprisoned on the grounds.

5. I knew that my grandfather's letters to my grandmother were destroyed, presumably because of her fear of leprosy. However, the painful nature of the two surviving letters to her make me believe that Edmond's letters were also destroyed to protect Teenie, Booz, and Claire herself from the emotional turmoil expressed in the letters and existing in the relationship between Edmond and Claire during much of his stay in Carville.

6. During the first half of the twentieth century, some patients built or cobbled together houses on the hospital grounds. They built them from scrap lumber they scavenged, materials they bought, or perhaps from kits ordered from Sears and Roebuck. These patients maintained residence in the institution but also frequently lived in or retreated to their cottages. When patients died or left Carville, their homes were passed along in informal, unregulated successions. My grandfather had such a cottage. After his death, my grandmother through her lawyer inquired about the property. Dr. Denney, the Medical Officer in Charge, indicated that he was unable to give them any information about the home. David Breaux, my companion and a reader of my work, suggests that because the houses were unofficial residences, they could neither be acknowledged nor denied by the administration.

7. The "What Cheer Club" was started by my grandfather, but named rather sardonically by another unidentified patient. The club was not without its political power struggles. Billy Lee, also a Carville patient, who according to some reports used a beer bottle as a gavel at meetings,

saw the potential that the club and canteen offered for personal gain, and he managed at some point to gain control of the club and the canteen funds. It was in part this disarray that led in the 1930s to the recreation of the "What Cheer Club" into the Patients Federation, an organization that became an active political force in the patient community until at least the closure of the federal hospital in 1998.

8. I am surprised at the rapid inception of the "What Cheer Club" and the canteen within four months of Edmond's entrance to Carville, but others have corroborated Stein's story that my grandfather founded both the canteen and the club. He was not the only one who quickly made a difference in the patient community. Stein himself was in Carville only two and a half months when he launched a patient newspaper, the *Sixty Six Star*. Perhaps when determination trumps lethargy, much can be accomplished quickly.

9. José Ramirez, a Hansen's disease patient in Carville in the 1960s and '70s, relates his own experience as a participant in such a training session for lay and medical personnel. He records feeling like a "slab of meat" on display when he was wheeled into the conference room in his robe and pajamas. The doctor in charge "grabbed my arm and with one swoop had me standing. He proceeded to remove my robe and pulled my pajama bottoms and boxer shorts down to my ankles. He was showing the audience open sores emphasizing what leprosy could do to the body if left untreated" (*Squint*, 63).

10. My grandfather was not the only patient involved in personal advocacy. Both Michelle Moran and Amy L. Fairchild make the case that Carville patients, as early as the 1890s, were active on their own behalf.

11. When she first read her father's medical records, my mother noted, "My father must have been a difficult patient."

12. Betty Martin, a patient peer of my grandfather, recalled the need for armed guards on visits home and she further noted that these guards were paid for by the patients or their families. A friend, Kevin McGowan, who has proofread this work, suggested that the guards accompanied the patients to protect them from fearful, ignorant outsiders, a possibility I had not considered.

CHAPTER 7

1. Albert may have written to his wife Sadie, from whom he was divorced in 1948, but none of these letters are in our collection. My mother and uncle always blamed Sadie for the divorce, but friends in Carville told me that Marie made it difficult for Albert and Sadie to visit alone. Sadie was not a leprosy patient, but she, too, was affected by the disease.

2. Carville had a patient's dining hall, but patients also fixed meals in their rooms on small hot plates.

3. At this time, Carville had an annual Christmas pageant that included a Nativity scene. I remember Daryl telling the story that one of the sisters, Sister Laura perhaps, used to have some whiskey behind stage as courage for the male patients. There are family pictures of Marie in elaborate spring performances with sets and a large cast. I do not know if such programs were in existence in the 1930s.

4. Amelie did not enter Carville when she first manifested symptoms; my mother's perception of Amelie's condition is that she had waited too long to seek treatment. Amelie's medical

records corroborate that view. Marie and Albert also waited until Marie was reported by authorities before going to the hospital. Neither Norbert nor Edmond was cured by being in the hospital, and all three of their siblings may have tried deferring the inevitable as long as they could, believing that a cure was not possible.

5. My mother recalls that in the week before he died, her grandfather, Terville, told her that he could feel the fish bone going down. His death was painful and unexpected. Even today, Lucie's family recalls that after Terville's death, fish was chewed by an adult before it was given to any of the children.

6. Mary Ruth, who came to Carville in 1939, remembered that the patients that year were disgruntled with the Medical Officer in Charge and used pressure to have him removed sometime in August.

7. It has never been clear to me who reported Albert, who was living in Opelousas at this time.

8. My grandmother still had a fear of HD. When my cousins and brothers began trying to explore the old family house in the late '50s, she had it torn down despite the fact that Dr. Johansen years earlier had declared that the house did not pose a threat. The cypress lumber from the house was either sold or given away, as were the furnishings. By the time the house was destroyed, Marie would have been unable to care for herself there, and Albert might have had no desire to live there either. Our family still owns the property.

9. The "three amigos" was the name José gave to these three older men: Darryl, Albert, and Milton, who meant so much to him in his life at Carville.

10. Albert and Marie were incarcerated in Carville in 1941. At the time of their mother's death in 1944, they were not able to get a pass to attend her funeral, but in the late 1950s, once leprosy was treatable, there was a move to discharge patients who no longer had active leprosy. My uncle's case record highlights the cognitive disconnect that occurred when decisions were made to discharge patients who had made their lives in the Carville community. According to 1958 records, Albert was a candidate for a discharge, but Marie was unable to care for herself, and Albert did not want to abandon his sister in Carville. He also had a reputation in the physical therapy department as a hard worker who was doing an excellent job and would be difficult to replace. Elsewhere, he was recognized for the great financial and social assistance he gave to patients in many situations. Ultimately Albert did remain in Carville until his death of heart failure in October 1977 but his was not the only such tragedy created for longtime Carville residents once leprosy was no longer a feared condition. This struggle to maintain the hospital and care for long term patients continued off and on for years. The hospital was finally closed in the late 1990s but patients who wished to do so were allowed to remain as long as they could maintain life for themselves. Once they were unable to care for themselves, they were transferred to a facility in Baton Rouge.

11. By this time, the federal government had provided housing for married couples so that they no longer had to build their own cottages or live separately in the male and female houses at the Carville institution.

12. This was in the late '60s or early '70s, but the stigma of Hansen's disease persisted. I remember in the mid-1970s excitedly telling Milton that I was going to college in San Antonio. He quietly said, "If you see me there, act like you don't recognize me."

13. Albert was a big man called "Tiny" by his friends in Carville and "Jelly" by his high school friends; despite his size he was always sharply dressed. Tanya Thommassie, a long time Carville employee, also remembered that Albert was always well dressed when he left the confines of Carville. I remember my own surprise when I discovered a picture of him not in a suit but in shirtsleeves.

CHAPTER 8

1. The works of Amy Shuman, Jane H. Hill, and Judith T. Irvin on entitlement were especially helpful.

2. After 1921, when the hospital became a federal institution, patients with Hansen's disease were required by federal law to be reported and incarcerated at the Carville institution. A letter regarding my grandfather's entrance to Carville explains that if he came of his own accord he would not be interdicted. Even into the mid-twentieth century, some unwilling patients were shackled to be brought to the hospital.

3. During the early years of the HIV/AIDS epidemic, there were similar condemnations and accusations. At one point, isolation of the sick, perhaps on an island somewhere was considered as an option—a fit protection for the good of others. My mother, usually quiet and non-committal, was vehement in her reaction to such proposals: "They *can't* do that!" She spoke from the depth of her experience.

4. I regret that family secrecy kept us mute for so long. I wish now that I had spoken to my Uncle Booz about his experiences because I sense that he, like my mother, may have spoken once his mother died. My grandmother never told her stories, but it was her silence that kept me curious and searching for my grandfather. I have come to believe that her silence, intentionally or unintentionally, kept the honor of my grandfather alive.

5. Marcia Gaudet, my nephew, and I were all working on Carville-related material.

6. Patricia Sawin's works on folk singer Bessie Eldreth suggests that the speech of others (reported speech) is used by women to say about themselves what they themselves would not or could not say. I believe my mother's stories reflect this same trope. Bessie used reported speech to offer the praise that others had given her without seeming to be bragging. My mother used the stories of others to relate her childhood experiences. Perhaps telling those stories in this reported fashion mitigated the pain that would have been unbearable had she told the stories in the first person.

7. Gaudet prefers the term counter narrative because it avoids the misconception that these are fictionalized accounts. I accept Gaudet's term.

8. See "The Art of Advocacy," by José Ramirez, on the website www.leprosysecrets.com for an account of Mr. Ramirez's efforts to advocate for truth about leprosy in contemporary movies.

9. My mother's surprising use of this all too common expletive is consistent with what W. E. H. Nicolaisen describes as a cultural registry, "the idea that people enact tradition when they perceive the situation to be appropriate" (255). For my mother, this was one time when this "tradition" was appropriate!

10. There were others in the Carville community who also told their stories. Marcia Gaudet's work chronicles and valorizes many of those. Stanley Stein, Betty Martin, D. J. Le Beaux, Johnny Harmon, and José Ramirez were others who wrote their own narratives.

11. At one point in the 1930s, the hospital chef used to publish the Sunday menu in the patient newsletter, the *Sixty Six Star*. One such menu advertised such culinary classics as crisp hearts of celery, California queen olives, stuffed eggs riverside, potage Neapolitan, chicken sauté a moringo, cauliflower with drawn butter, new potatoes in crème, and steamed rice. The meal sounded enticing but it was still an institutional dinner.

Works Cited

Archives. Gillis W. Long National Hansen's Disease Center, Carville, Louisiana. (Much of this material has been transferred to the archives of the Daughters of Charity in St. Louis, Mo., and will be transferred to the provincial archives in Bethesda, Md.)

Bennett, Gillian. "Narratives as Expository Discourse." *Journal of American Folklore* 99 (1986): 415–434.

Bok, Sissela. *Secrets: On the Ethics of Concealment and Revelation*. New York: Pantheon Books, 1982.

Breaux, David. Personal conversations, 1999–2012.

Carruth, Cathy, ed. *Trauma: Explorations in Memory*. Baltimore: Johns Hopkins University Press, 1991.

Elwood, Julia, ed. *Known Simply to the World as Carville . . . 100 Years*. Carville, La: Department of Health and Human Services. U.S. Public Health Service, Gillis W. Long National Hansen's Disease Center, 1994.

Elwood, Julia, and Ray Elwood. Email messages with the author, Spring 2011.

Fairchild, Amy L. "Leprosy, Domesticity, and Patient Protest: The Social Context of a Patients' Rights Movement in Mid-Century America." *Journal of Social History* 39:4 (Summer 2006), 1011–1043.

Frank, Arthur W. *The Wounded Storyteller: Body, Illness, and Ethics*. Chicago: University of Chicago Press, 1995.

Gaudet, Marcia. *Carville: Remembering Leprosy in America*. Jackson: University Press of Mississippi, 2004.

Goffman, Erving. *Stigma: Notes on the Management of Spoiled Identity*. New York: Touchstone Books, 1986.

Harmon, Johnny P. *King of the Microbes: The Autobiography of Johnny Harmon*. 4th printing. Baton Rouge, 1998., n.p.

Hill, Jane H., and Judith T. Irvine. *Responsibility and Evidence in Oral Discourse*. Cambridge: Cambridge University Press, 1992.

Hirsch, Marianne. *Family Frames: Photography, Narrative and Postmemory*. Cambridge and London: Harvard University Press, 1997.

———. "Projected Memory: Holocaust Photography in Personal and Public Fantasy." In *Acts of Memory: Cultural Recall in the Present*. Edited by Mieke Bal, Jonathan Crewe, and Leo Spitzer. Hanover and London: University Press of New England, 1999, 3–23.

Jung, Carl G. *Collected Works of C. G. Jung*. Vol. 4, *Freud and Psychoanalysis*. Translated by R. F. C. Hull. Princeton: Princeton University Press, 1961.

———. Vol. 16, *The Practice of Psychotherapy: Essays on the Psychology of the Transference and Other Subjects*, 2nd ed. Translated by R. F. C. Hull. Princeton: Princeton University Press, 1966.

Kolb, Carolyn. *New Orleans Magazine*, November 2005, 106.

Landry, Albert, Amelie Landry, Edmond Landry, Marie Landry, and Norbert Landry. From medical records in possession of the author.

Landry Letters from Carville. Private collection of letters and artifacts, 1908–1960. Landry Letters from Carville, LLC. Used by permission.

Lawless, Elaine J. *Women Escaping Violence: Empowerment through Narrative*. Columbia: University of Missouri Press, 2001.

LeBeaux, D. J. *Love Me, Somebody*. New York: Vantage Press, 1985.

Manes, Christopher Lee. "Regardez." Master's thesis. University of Louisiana at Lafayette, 2003.

Manes, Claire. "In His Own Hand: The Correspondence of Edmond G. Landry from Carville, Louisiana." *Louisiana Folklore Miscellany* 20: 2010: 51–61. (A version of this article was presented at the Louisiana Folklore Conference, Lafayette, La., in 2003.)

Manes, Leonide Landry. Ongoing conversations with the author, 1998–2007.

Martin, Betty. *Miracle at Carville*. EdIted by Evelyn Wells. Garden City, NY: Doubleday, 1950.

———. *No One Must Ever Know*. New York: Doubleday, 1959.

Mary Ruth. Requested identification, Carville resident. Personal conversations and interviews, Carville, Louisiana, 1979–2003.

Moran, Michelle T. *Colonizing Leprosy: Imperialism and the Politics of Public Health in the United States*. Chapel Hill: University of North Carolina Press, 2007.

Mullen, Patrick B. "A Traditional Storyteller in Changing Contexts." In *"And Other Neighborly Names" Social Process and Cultural Image in Texas Folklore*. Edited by Richard Bauman and Roger D. Abrahams. Austin: University of Texas Press, 1981: 266–79.

Nelson, Hilde Lindemann. *Damaged Identities, Narrative Repair*. Ithaca: Cornell University Press, 2001.

Nicolaisen, W. E. H. "Cultural Register." In *Encyclopedia of American Folklore*, Vol. 1. Edited by Simon Bronner. New York: M. E. Sharp, 2006.

Radner, Joan Newton. *Feminist Messages: Coding in Women's Folk Culture*. Chicago: University of Illinois Press, 1993.

Ramirez, José, Jr. *Squint: My Journey with Leprosy*. Jackson: University Press of Mississippi, 2009.

———. Emails to author 2011–present.

Sawin, Patricia. *Listening for a Life: a Dialogic Ethnography of Bessie Eldreth through Her Songs and Stories*. Logan: Utah State University Press, 2004.

———"'Right Here Is a Good Christian Lady': Reported Speech in Personal Narratives." *Text and Performances Quarterly* 12.3 (1992): 193–211.

Schexnyder, Elizabeth. Curator National Hansen's Disease Museum. Carville, Louisiana. Ongoing support and conversations with the author, 2006–2012.

Shuman, Amy. *Other People's Stories: Entitlement Claims and the Critique of Empathy.* Urbana and Chicago: University of Illinois Press, 2005.

———. "'Outa My Face': Entitlement and Authoritative Discourse." In *Responsibility and Evidence in Oral Discourse.* Edited by Jane H. Hill and Judith T. Irvine. Cambridge: Cambridge University Press, 1992, 135–150.

Stahl, Sandra Dolby. "A Literary Folkloristic Methodology for the Study of Meaning in Personal Narrative." *Journal of Folklore Research* 22:1 (1985): 45–69.

———. *Literary Folkloristics and the Personal Narrative.* Bloomington: Indiana University Press, 1989.

———. "The Personal Narrative as Folklore." *Journal of the Folklore Institute* 14.1–2 (1977): 9–31.

Sixty Six Star 1931–1934. In-house publication at the United States Public Health Services Hospital #66. Archived in Carville, Louisiana. Copy in private collection of author.

Stein, Stanley, with Lawrence G. Blockman. *Alone No Longer.* New York: Funk and Wagnalls, 1963.

Taussig, Michael. *Defacement: Public Secret and the Labor of the Negative.* Stanford: Stanford University Press, 1999.

Truman, Richard W. *Los Angeles Times*, April 27, 2011.

Wilhelm, John, and Sally Squires. *Triumph at Carville A Tale of Leprosy in America.* DVD. The Wilhelm Group, 2005.

Index